Evolutionary Meditation Science

from stress reduction to enlightenment

by Jason Augustus Newcomb

Evolutionary Meditation Science

from stress reduction to enlightenment

by Jason Augustus Newcomb

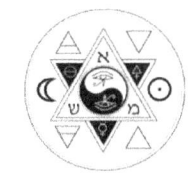

The New Hermetics Press
Sarasota, FL

First published in 2020 by
The New Hermetics Press
P. O. Box 18111
Sarasota, FL 34276
www.newhermetics.com

Copyright © 2020 Jason Augustus Newcomb

All rights reserved. No part of this publication may be reproduced or transmitted in any form or by any means, electronic or mechanical, including photocopying, recording, or by any information storage and retrieval system, without permission in writing from The New Hermetics Press. Reviewers may quote brief passages.

ISBN: 978-1-63118-393-5

Cover Design and typesetting by Fr∴ E. I. A. E.
Editorial assistance by Fr∴ I. T. I. F. E. L.

26 25 24 23 22 21 20 19
8 7 6 5 4 3 2 1

DEDICATED TO
Swami Vivekananda

OTHER BOOKS BY JASON AUGUSTUS NEWCOMB

Nonfiction:

21st Century Mage (Weiser Books, 2002)
The New Hermetics (Weiser Books, 2004)
Sexual Sorcery (Weiser Books, 2005)

The Book of Magick Power
Practical Enochian Magick: A Manual for the New Hermetics Adept
The Advanced Adept Manual and Workbook
Conjuring the Goetia Spirits: A Simple Advanced Key (limited edition)
The New Hermetics Equinox Journal Vol. 1-5
Dodekameron
A Modern User's Guide to Trithemius' "Art of Drawing Spirits into Crystals"
And many more!

Fiction:

The Brotherhood of Light and Darkness

CONTENTS

Read this First	9
PART 1 - MEDITATION THEORY	
Meditation Models, Ancient and Modern	13
The Thrupple of Attention	31
Lucid vs. Sluggish Relaxation	36
Attentional Reward vs. Distraction Punishment	38
Foveal vs. Peripheral Awareness	40
Habituation vs. Seeking Novelty	41
Beliefs, Opinions and Preferences	42
Breathing, Relaxation and Your Body	43
Stumbling blocks in Meditation Practice	47
How to Approach Meditation Skillfully	51
The Five Basic Levels of Meditative Skill	53
The Four Basic Focal Absorption Stages	56
PART 2 - MEDITATION TOOLS AND PARTS	
The Preliminary Stretch	63
Posture	64
Recollection of Intent	68
Breathing	70
Relaxing	71
The Central Practice	72
Elevating Emotions	73
Future Pacing	76
Sharing Benefits	77
Some Meta Tools	78
PART 3 - MEDITATION PRACTICES	
Focus	83
Mantra	87
Bhakti	89
Breath	92
Mindful	94
Inquiry	97
Deep Pranayama	105
Fast Pranayama	106
1:4:2 Pranayama	108
Breathing Visualization Patterns	110
Conclusion	113

Read this First

This book is a practical instruction in how training consciousness can improve health, well-being and even lead to enlightenment with practical methods based on the scientific research available to support these claims. I want you to start meditating, and for your meditation practice to be something you enjoy, and something that is transformative.

I am going to assume that you have picked up this book because you are one of the millions of people who have been becoming interested in meditation in the last few years.

You are looking for a technique to feel more relaxed, reduce stress and maybe some of the other health benefits that have been credited to meditation in the last few years. Some of these include pain management, reducing blood pressure, easing depression, weight loss, improving the immune system, ending insomnia, addiction recovery, and so on and so on. Meditation seems to have a very positive effect on these symptoms. It is a real panacea, and it is fairly easy to do.

But truthfully, suggesting that the best use for meditation is to help with insomnia or anxiety is like saying that the best use for a motorcycle is to make loud noises. Yes, motorcycles are great at being loud, but they are made for driving around. Yes, meditation will make people feel better, but it was made to help people see through the illusions of ego and to become free from suffering. The purpose of meditation is to become enlightened.

There are a number of popular meditation movements that have been coming in and out of vogue for the last few decades: Transcendental Meditation, Vipassana, Centering Prayer, Mindfulness Based Stress Relief, Tibetan Vajrayana etc. All of them have claimed to be the best methods, and all can cost hefty amounts of money to learn. But truthfully they all are just different approaches to precisely the same goal, and they are all easy to do once you understand the core principles more fully.

Following the simple instructions in this book you are going to learn how to meditate extremely well, quite quickly, and you will discover the health benefits for yourself, but you are also going to learn to see the world in an enlightened way.

I want to give you a fun book that is easy to read, easy to use, and teaches you to become enlightened. I also want you to know that what I am saying is supported by hard clinical research. I'm going to try not to say much that isn't supported by credible research or well established fact.

So, who am I, and why did I create this book? My background is in applied consciousness studies. I have been teaching meditation and altered states of consciousness for almost thirty years. I used to think I knew a lot about the subject, and then in the last decade I learned some new things about the topic and realized I still had a lot to learn. This little book is some of what I've learned.

I am not a part of any religion. I am not promoting any religion or religious organization. I am just going to teach you how to meditate so effectively that you are going to become an enlightened being if you want to. You can be an enlightened Christian, Muslim, Jew, Hindu, Buddhist, Atheist or any other label you prefer. Or you may decide to drop the labels. Or you may decide all the labels describe you.

You don't have to be enlightened either. You can just rev the motor of the motorcycle if that's what you want.

I have also created a series of audio recordings based upon the practices in this book so if you want to make the process incredibly easy you can just go grab one or more of those recordings. But keep reading.

This book is intentionally fairly short and to the point. Meditation is a simple and straightforward process. You do not need to read thousands of pages of spiritual mumbo-jumbo to learn meditation or to become enlightened. The important thing to do is to meditate regularly, and to meditate in a way that is going to produce the fruit of enlightenment. That is the aim of this little book.

There will be some metaphysical jargon along the way too, although I am not going to hang important facts only on jargon pointing at other jargon. If there is some foreign word that you don't understand it is safe to ignore it. It is probably there so that more fussy readers will see that I know what I'm talking about. If you are confused about any of the instructions please come to one of my many free meditation classes both online and in person. I am always happy to answer questions.

What is Meditation?

Meditation means a lot of different things to a lot of different people. On the one hand it is spiritual techniques used by monks, yogis and religious practitioners. But nowadays there are many mindfulness techniques taught by therapists and doctors.

Could all of these people really be teaching the same thing? The truth is that there is a good deal of variety in what they teach and how they teach it, as well as why they are teaching it. But the central core of meditation is really all one thing.

For the purposes of this book meditation is ***the act of focusing the attention on a single object, and maintaining a present awareness of what we are focusing upon.*** This definition covers all forms of meditation, although some forms of meditation may add another aspect or two.

For instance, more religious forms of meditation would add a necessary sense of divine love and devotion. Some Hatha Yoga practices might involve moving inner energies, controlling the breath and other specifics. We will learn a bit more about both of these matters later in this book. Nevertheless, the essence of meditation is the act of focusing attention on some object in present awareness.

Despite sounding rather simple, this act is of course much easier said than done, even in its most simple form. Take a moment and stare at the black dot on the next page. Simply place your whole attention on the dot and don't think about anything but the dot. Try to experience the dot fully, and keep your whole attention on the dot.

●

If you are a normal person, your mind started wandering within ten seconds or so. Our brains are conditioned by nature to search for new information, to look for prey or to avoid predators. It is natural for the animal brain to seek for new information rather than fixating on a black dot.

Meditation mastery is also based upon another natural occurrence in consciousness, but uses it in a special way. When our ancestors were out exploring in nature, at the moment a predator or prey animal moved into their awareness, they naturally shifted consciousness into a state of absolute attention. The sense of the ego dissolved in a need for immediate action. Meditation trains you to enter this state of attention without the stress and anxiety of the sympathetic nervous system flooding the body with fight or flight chemicals.

We see a similar awareness in the flow states of athletes, artists, musicians and writers who lose themselves in the absolute focus of their work. Many, while staying in a state of absolute present awareness, feel as if they are somehow just the vessel, and not the doer of the work at all.

A gentle training of the consciousness allows this deep level of awareness to develop in states of relaxation rather than tension.

The basic action of meditation is simply repeatedly returning to the present moment every time attention wanders. You focus upon the meditation object, and then fairly quickly attention gets lost in something extraneous. When you notice, you return consciousness to the meditation object. Then distracting things come up in your mind again and again you return to the meditation object.

Over time, the mind picks up the habit, and attention remains more and more centered on the object. First you will notice that despite distractions coming up, the distraction is noticed more and more quickly. Then as you develop, you will find yourself maintaining your focus and even though distractions continue to arise, you will continue to keep the meditation object in awareness even in the midst of distraction. Then, eventually you will be able to rest on the meditation object, completely absorbed.

When this complete focus is accomplished without any strain or exertion our consciousness becomes flooded with a sense of joy and ecstasy. Very often we see lights, hear strange sounds or feel flows of energy and even the presence of spiritual helpers. These sorts of mystical experience have been described across the world by basically every culture, though filtered through the beliefs of each culture. But this isn't the end goal of meditation. It is just a step in the process.

This repeated action of returning your awareness to your meditation object also has a secondary benefit in your life in general after you have been doing it for a while you will notice that when you enter into states of consciousness that are less productive or useful your mind will automatically start to return you to the present moment and this will give you an opportunity to react more skillfully.

This doesn't mean that meditation will automatically make you less reactive but it will make you more aware that you are being reactive, and over time you will find yourself being nicer and more centered. This is not necessarily the main aim of meditation but it is a beneficial effect that you will observe. In fact this may be the main effect that scientists presently observe and appreciate in meditation. However we are going to be traveling a bit further along than most science based programs.

We are scientifically seeking enlightenment. How meditation does this and the reasons you would want this will be revealed as we continue forward.

What is Enlightenment?

This topic is one that causes a lot of confusion. Early European translators of Vedic and Buddhist texts used the term "enlightenment" to describe the transcendent goal of a meditative practice but the translation is not very descriptive or appropriate. The Enlightenment in Europe of the 17th and 18th centuries meant a new intellectual freedom that gave birth to the scientific method, modern political democracy, and new more personalized artistic expressions. This is not really what the enlightenment from meditation is about, although the two are not in opposition. But they are hardly even related, other than through the linguistic convention of the early translators.

Two of the most common Sanskrit terms we find for enlightenment in the ancient texts are *moksha* and *nirvana* (or *nibbana* in Pali). Additionally, a term used most frequently in the *Yoga Sutras* is *kaivalya*. It translates to something like "isolation," and represents awareness separated from the world of ego illusions. *Moksha* translates more closely to "freedom" and represents freedom from the ego mind in the transcendent awareness of the divine Self. *Nirvana* means something like "snuffed out" and represents the cessation of the tendencies toward craving and aversion as the ego is transcended.

In the Christian mysticism of Paul in his second letter to the Galatians we see, "It is no longer I who live, but Christ who lives in me." So, we see the same sort of ego loss in the Christian who unites with God in the blissful union of complete devotion.

The connecting point of these different terms and philosophies is *a consciousness in being that operates completely without the inherent suffering of a self-centered awareness separate from the rest of existence.*[1]

This experience is not really all that far off. In meditative absorption you will have the experience of this way of being. So, you will experience enlightenment as a "state of consciousness," in the next few months if you begin a regular practice today and follow the simple suggestions for smart and successful practice covered throughout this book. This state will be temporary at first, as you will go back to old patterns that are more familiar when you are just getting started. Over time, it will become more and more who you are- an enlightened being.

---

[1] This could also be called "Union with God," but it must be understood that the vast majority of religious meditators see the highest form of the divine as being entirely without form or attributes and so in actuality indistinguishable and inseparable from pure awareness itself.

PART 1 – MEDITATION THEORY

Meditation Models, Ancient and Modern

Meditation has nothing specifically to do with Buddhism, Yoga or any other eastern religious movement. There are numerous practices of meditation within Christianity, Judaism and Islam, although they have often been kept hidden behind the doors of monasteries and nunneries. Meditation is described by ancient Greek philosophers, Mesopotamian and Egyptian priests, and has been a part of our evolving cultures for thousands of years. Meditation doesn't really have anything to do with religion or spirituality at all. Meditation is a technology for focusing and looking at consciousness directly to uncover its essential nature. Many practitioners of meditation have been secular atheists throughout the centuries. There are meditation practices that can be traced to virtually every culture and religion, and all of them fit within the basic descriptions above.

This being said, meditation has always been a central spiritual tool for many thousands of years, and has often been preserved only for the most serious practitioners and devotees of spirituality. But in the twenty-first century it has been taken up by the health industry as a cure all for many of our deep-seated mental problems. But setting aside these two poles of deep spirituality and health fad, meditation can help us with the much more basic problem that we have as a species which is a basic dissatisfaction with our existence and a fundamental lack of knowledge about who we are and what we are. Meditation offers us access to the same insights as religious giants, mental giants and heroes of the past. Meditation conducted correctly will increase your intelligence, your stamina, your confidence, and your sense of comfort in your skin.

Religious Models for Meditation
Buddhism

The vast majority of meditation techniques and principles being taught today here in the United States and Europe come from Buddhism. Buddhism is a complex subject that contains many entirely separate religions and here in the West we largely to don't distinguish between these all that well. There is a huge difference between the Tantric

Vajrayana Buddhism of Tibet, the Nichiren Buddhism of Japan and the Theravada Buddhism of Sri Lanka and Burma. These religions are extremely different from one another and while they all share the term Buddhism and have as their central teaching figure the Buddha, the teachings are very dissimilar. We are not going concern ourselves greatly with divergent matters of theology or religious philosophy. In this book we are concerned with the practicalities of meditation. However a few words must be said about Buddhism and other religions because they play an influential part in the development of the techniques of meditation.

Not all forms of Buddhism give an equal place to meditation or practice it in the same way. For instance there is a pretty wide difference between the Zen Buddhism of Japan and the Jhana practiced by Thai forest monks despite the linguistic relationship of the words. Like a game of telephone that has taken place over 2500 years the ideas and practices of Buddhism have shifted dramatically as it has spread across the globe.

The westernized versions of Buddhism that we get imported to us in Europe and the Americas are very different in tone from those of practitioners elsewhere. As a culture we tend to be quite atheistic because we have distanced ourselves from our own religious roots in Christianity in favor of modern science so those aspects of Buddhism that are particularly religious in tone tend to get rooted out of American and European Buddhist practice.

The ideas of reincarnation and beings in other realms of existence, psychic and magical powers attributed to the Buddha and his students, and really all metaphysical matters have largely been washed out of Buddhism for most practicing Western Buddhists. And when scientists encounter these Buddhists and try to learn meditation techniques for medical purposes even more gets taken out so that what was once a method for experiencing a divine awakening just becomes an exotic relaxation technique for improving one's mood. What you are going to be learning in these pages is influenced by traditional Buddhist practice and the innovations of modern meditation.

Yoga

Yoga has become extremely popular over the past couple of decades. Much like Buddhism, the impression we have in the west is an extremely watered down and distorted picture of what Yoga is really about. Most people just see Yoga as a series of postures used to stretch and get a "Yoga Butt." However, Yoga is a broad term that describes many different types of spiritual practice, most of which have nothing to do with stretching or posing. Yoga means union, and the many different types of Yoga are all means of establishing union with divine consciousness. While there are many more types of Yoga than we can discuss in this space, they are most frequently divided into two possible lists of four general practices.

Mantra Yoga – the use of sacred sounds to unite with the divine
Hatha Yoga – the use of energies and force to unite with the divine
Laya Yoga – the use of dissolution practices to unite with the divine
Raja Yoga – the use of dharana, dhyana and samadhi (meditation) to unite with the divine

-or-

Karma Yoga – the use of action and activity to unite with the divine
Bhakti Yoga – the use of devotion to unite with the divine
Jnana Yoga – the use of knowledge (often associated with self-inquiry) to unite with the divine
Raja Yoga – also dharana, dhyana and samadhi

Today, what most people associate with the term Yoga is just one version of one preliminary part of Hatha Yoga or Raja Yoga. It is the "asana" or postural component of these multipart systems which usually have either six or eight components involving posture, breathing, mental focus and meditation. For completeness it should also be mentioned that the postures most often associated with Yoga have nearly nothing to do with its deeper components. Most of what we call Yoga today is really a very modern twentieth century health movement that combines elements from European fitness and dance with Indian acrobatics and contortionism.

Traditional Yoga philosophy is dualistic in nature. Matter and consciousness are distinct entities, called respectively *Prakriti* and *Purusha*. This makes no practical impact on the specific techniques of meditation, but it means that the traditional goal of Yoga itself is actually closer to the aim of contemplative Christianity than that of Buddhism. The Yogi is attempting to unite with the divine, sometimes called *Isvara*, rather than to uncover a non-dual experience. While this is really quibbling over details that are not going to impact your practice at this time, I feel it is important to realize that much of the "body positive" aspects of Yoga are actually foreign infusions from our western culture that are not really a part of the original Yoga systems at all, which tend to be quite antagonistic toward the body, placing value only on the divine, and moving consciousness away from matter, into the divine consciousness.

The earliest written instruction we have for Yoga meditation is Pantanjali's *Yoga Sutras* which is possibly as much as 3000 years old[2] and describes, among other things, an eight part process of establishing union with the divine consciousness. Yoga is also described in *Bhagavad Gita* and in the *Upanishads,* and a large amount of practical literature on the subject began to appear in the fifteenth or sixteenth century of our common era. Again however, very little of this literature has anything to do with most Yoga classes.

While Yoga possesses a lot of meditation techniques, most of these are not well described in the existing popular literature, and you will almost never find them in a Yoga class. If there is any meditation in your average Yoga class, it is much more likely to be based upon Buddhist mindfulness practices. This is not really a huge problem, since as I keep mentioning, meditation is a pretty universal phenomenon. However, the confusion often creates misunderstandings about the purpose and practicalities of many techniques within Hatha practice. The *Yoga Sutras* of Patanjali list most of the six main meditation styles we will discuss later.

There are also other "branded" types of Yoga, most of which are fairly modern creations, while based upon older traditions. Amongst these are

---

[2] Although much of modern scholarship tends to view it as significantly younger.

the so-called Kriya Yoga,[3] Vinyasa Yoga, and Kundalini Yoga. In this book you will be learning several techniques directly adapted from traditional Yoga meditational practices such as *pranayama, dharana, trataka* and other more advanced techniques.

Kundalini and Chakras

Kundalini is an interesting topic within the field of meditation, as her awakening is often held to be very central to success in various schools of spiritual development, yet there are a lot of different opinions about what Kundalini even is. To some she is a goddess, to others the basic energy of life or the force of consciousness evolution. To some she is a dangerous unbalancing force that should be avoided unless you are seeking trouble. However, whether she is the core energy of the universe, or of humanity, or the goddess within us, or anything else, the more you look into meditation systems that derive from the Indian subcontinent in one way or another, the more you see her name coming up.

The earliest references to her in the Indian Upanishads and older Tantric literature make it clear that she is a goddess. But these very same philosophical systems don't always make a clear distinction between things that are inside consciousness and in things the outer world, so it is often hard to pin down precisely what is being said. Further, one of the names of the goddess is *Shakti*, which means power, and so could easily be describing a force or energy as much as a personified being.

By the time we reach Hatha Yoga literature in the 13th century CE, we clearly see Kundalini equated with a force or energy dormant in the body, while still retaining qualities as a goddess at the same time. This energy/goddess is awakened by certain physical and psychological actions and her awakening is the cause of, or at least precipitates, enlightenment or liberation.

Moving to the practical matters that you are likely encounter, there are a lot of sensations that come up when we are meditating and some people

---

[33] That version popularized by Paramahansa Yogananda, not the Kriya Yoga described by Patanjali. The two seem to have virtually nothing in common.

identify these with Kundalini. There are other names for the energetic experiences that come up in meditation such as *prana,* or other "inner winds" or *vayus, chi, orgone, vril,* The Descent of the Holy Spirit, and dozens of others in many different cultures. Some people say that when Kundalini awakens it is a shocking and transforming experience that is unmistakable. Others say that Kundalini awakening is a very subtle and beautiful experience. Perhaps it is different for different people.

It doesn't really matter for our purposes and we are going to just refer to all of these sorts of phenomena as inner energy movement experiences. You are most likely going to experience these sooner or later, and expecting to do so will make it easier. Some of the more breathing centered techniques that you are going to be learning are, in their classic forms, really focused on awakening this Kundalini. You will experience very profound energy experiences with these techniques.

You also may experience powerful energy phenomena during any other meditation techniques in this book. Very often these sensations are centered in particular centralized areas of the body. These areas are often called chakras, and you will most likely have energetic experiences related to these areas as well. In particular the areas at the center of your chest and the center of your forehead, the so-called "heart chakra" and "third eye" chakra will often produce all sorts of ecstatic and profound feelings, visions and experiences. Just allow these things to happen as they do. There is no real need to attach a complex metaphysical theory to the experience.

Some people say these sorts of experiences are dangerous because they are often powerful and even sometimes painful. Driving in your automobile without a safety belt is dangerous, and frankly riding in your automobile at all in general is dangerous. I don't think having a difficult energy experience in your own consciousness is really something to fear. If you do fear it you may wish to stay away from these practices. If you have a history of psychological problems of course I recommend talking to a medical professional before doing any practice whatsoever.

Christian Contemplation, Kabbalah and Sufism

Christianity also has a very long history of meditation techniques though they have often been called contemplation or silent prayer. This too has been becoming somewhat more popular in the past few decades however these meditation techniques can be traced back to the very beginning of the Christian movement in the first years of our modern calendar. These techniques also do not differ very much from those of Yoga or Buddhism.

Islam and Judaism, particularly in their more esoteric forms of Kabbalah and Sufism, also have meditation techniques and again these do not differ in any great way from the meditation practices anywhere else. Meditation is a basic universal religious practice. In mystical Judaism, the practice of meditation is most frequently called *hitbodedut,* which can be translated as self-isolation. The Sanskrit term *kaivalya,* a word for the goal of Yoga, translates to the same thing. In both cases the goal is to be alone with the divine consciousness that is ever present in the deepest recesses of awareness. The Arabic term *muraqabah,* which translated as "to observe," has an identical purpose in Sufism, to center awareness on the divine.

It is really only the descriptions of the religious results that differ within each culture. A Christian or Jew says they rest in the love of union with God. A Buddhist says that they have ceased to suffer in the bliss of *nirvana.* A yogi says they have accomplished *jivanmukti* and are one with the *atman* or *purusha.* And maybe these results are somewhat different from each other, influenced by the expectations of the practitioner. Maybe you want one of these results and you don't want one of the others. It doesn't really matter because the techniques are essentially the same either way.

The key to it all is that you engage the "thrupple of attention"[4] upon an object and experience it completely without analyzing or labeling it with your ego. The Christian writer from the 13th century calls this engaging with the "cloud of forgetting" to lose yourself and enter into the "cloud

---

[4] This term will be explained very soon.

of unknowing" to become one with God in pure love. But the technique is to repeat the word "God" over and over again in the mind while putting your attention toward a loving conception of God. A Yogi says she accomplishes liberation by quieting the *chitta* or mind stuff, entering *samadhi* and finally *moksha* disappearing into *purusha* or *atman*. But the technique is to repeat the mantra over and over while giving yourself over in devotion to *Isvara*. The Buddhist says they accomplished *nirvana* or *nibbana*. The technique involves repeating the word "Earth, Earth, Earth," over and over while visualizing the element everywhere, engaging the attention single pointedly, until you enter the unconditioned, unborn. I could list one hundred slightly varying techniques and point out how ultimately they are doing the same thing but hopefully you get my drift and we can move on.

Scientific Models for Meditation
Freud, Jung and the Unconscious

Sigmund Freud MD proposed that many of our personal problems come from complexes outside of our conscious awareness in what he came to call the unconscious mind. His student Carl Jung MD expanded the concept into what he called the collective unconscious which expanded modern psychology more and more into the realms previously occupied by religious and spiritual pursuits.

Today, most psychology is practiced with the use of various psychoactive chemicals attempting to balance out the neurology, rather than engaging with subjective material in consciousness much at all. However, modern psychology really began with the study of altered states of consciousness and its therapeutic effects. Early psychiatrists frequently used hypnosis or "animal magnetism" to cure problems for many difficult patients. Eventually analysis and various theories of the unconscious began to predominate and the idea of catharsis through recognition of material previously outside of awareness became the standard therapeutic tool. And then pharmaceuticals became even more popular.

The theory of an unconscious aspect of the human mind has gone in and out of fashion over the decades, but it cannot be denied that there are parts of our consciousness to which we do not always have access.

Chances are you are not aware of the sensation of your arm folded over your armpit and yet when I mention it you realize it is always there. And further you can realize that cellular repair and blood flow in the same armpit are constantly being managed by a part of your brain and nervous system over which you have very little awareness or control ever. Meditation offers a simple and powerful method of opening up to the totality of awareness, including this unconscious material, and it is in this fusion between the known and the unknown that creates a deeper awareness of reality as well as profound energy experiences or experiences of beings and other worlds. Enlightenment is found in this material, letting go of our preconceptions and illusions and experiencing the entirety of your consciousness.

The experience of this unconscious material can be both a blessing and a challenge. It is very often necessary to deal with "stuff," as a result of regular sitting practice. This is not the purpose of meditation, but it is sometimes a side effect. Along with troubling experiences you will also open up to greater resources within yourself and a greater understanding of very positive aspects of your consciousness that have remained dormant outside of your awareness. But if you are prone to psychological issues, it might be useful to consult your physician about your meditation practice so that any challenges can be handled with support.

Altered States of Consciousness

Meditation is an altered state of consciousness. Actually, it is the skillful use of several different altered states of consciousness, mastered and achieved sequentially and intentionally over time. However, we humans experience many kinds of altered states of consciousness all the time. When we get really lost in a good book or movie, when we get frightened in the dark to the point in which we lose our breath, or drink too much wine at dinner, in each of these cases we are entering into an altered state of consciousness.

Altered states can be anything from mood changes to dramatic personality shifts, sometimes even causing amnesia. Profound altered states can bring us visions, hallucinations and ecstasies, and even occasionally fearful material. Whether mundane or dramatic, everyone experiences these shifts.

These shifts are natural, and have been being observed and utilized in various ways for thousands of years. One of the primary ways is, of course, in creating spiritual experiences in ourselves and others. Modern science has had a rather tempestuous relationship with these states, because they are invisible and ephemeral, making them less desirable than many topics science usually tries to understand. But since they are an undeniable component of human experience, researchers have been studying them in earnest for the last few decades.

The Autonomic Nervous System

One of the ways in which we understand altered states is through changes in the autonomic nervous system. The autonomic nervous system runs the unconscious systems of our body such as our heart rate, respiration, fluids, the function of our organs and all the processes that keep us alive and healthy when we are busy over thinking other things.

We divide the autonomic nervous system into three components, the sympathetic, the parasympathetic and the enteric nervous system. Broadly, the first of these is often called the "fight or flight" system, the second the "rest and digest," and the third the "abdominal brain." The sympathetic system is active when we are stimulated by immediate concerns, dangers or problem solving. The parasympathetic system activates the balance and healing in our bodies when we are relaxed or pleasantly stimulated. The enteric system controls our digestive and other bodily systems.

Research on meditation has shown definitively that it increases the calming activity of the parasympathetic system, stimulating relaxation ad cellular repair, and it is this benefit that has produced the most support from the scientific community since it has a clear physiological benefit. This relaxation produces many of the health benefits credited to meditation including lowering stress, lowering blood pressure, eliminating headaches, and releasing some the negative effects of our hectic lives.

Brain Research

In the 1950s, neurosurgeon Wilder Penfield MD discovered that by electrically stimulating the brain tissue of the temporal lobe of his patients he could produce vivid hallucinations, out-of-body experiences and even encounters with God. As fascinating as this research was, not many people have access to someone who can open up their skulls and shock their brain tissues with electricity for spiritual purposes. However, Dr. Penfield did discover that most mystical experiences he produced related to stimulation of the sylvan fissure between the frontal and temporal lobes of the brain. This may someday yield further insight into these sorts of experiences.

More recently Andrew Newberg MD has conducted extensive neurological research into the areas of the brain that activate during meditation and enlightenment types of experiences, and even offers some practical advice in his book *How Enlightenment Changes Your Brain* largely focuses on aha! moments rather than a regular meditation practice as a gradual process of insight and transformation, so there are some significant limits to the usefulness of his advice. Knowing where your brain lights up when you are experiencing enlightenment does not necessarily help in getting into the states conducive to real and lasting transformative change, but the work is highly interesting.

Other research has indicated long term differences in the brain patterns of meditators and non-meditators which seem to indicate that over time our ability to deal with stress, improved decision making, creative thinking and other benefits are clearly associated with meditation. Much more research needs to be done in this area, but there is little doubt that meditation will be shown to have a very and measurable effect on the human organism.

Brainwaves

Another way in which researchers analyze the changes of consciousness is through different patterns of brainwaves that dominate during different states when a subject is connected to an electro-encephalograph (EEG) machine. Consciousness is a very fluid and elusive thing, so this model is a bit simplistic, and all of these states can somewhat blend into one another It is not possible to strictly say that one thing is always this and another that. Still, it is useful as a way of classifying general experiences. All of the brainwaves appear all the time, but certain ones predominate during certain experiences.

Beta – brainwave frequency: 14 to 30 cycles per second

These are the kind of brainwaves that are most observed by an EEG machine when we are in an active and alert state of mind. This is a state of outer awareness in which we are focused on what is going on around us.

Alpha – brainwave frequency: 8 to 13 cycles per second

These are the brainwave patterns observed when a person is deeply relaxed and focused inwardly. It's often called the light trance. This is the state we are often in when watching TV or a movie, meditating and relaxing, doing yoga, or driving long distances on the highway. Many of us spend a lot of time in this state.

Theta – brainwave frequency: 4 to 7 cycles per second

This is the state associated with extreme relaxation and the deeper trance states of advanced meditation or deep hypnosis. It is sometimes called the "hypnagogic state." This is that usually brief time between waking and sleeping when images, sounds and mini-dreams seem to come into your mind of their own volition. When you focus your consciousness in this state you can have those mystical "peak experiences" associated with illumination and transcendence. You may also be actually asleep in this state. You usually do not have much awareness of your body in the Theta State, although you may feel vibrations, ripples or slowly spinning sensations.

Delta – brainwave frequency: .5 to 3 cycles per second

This is the state of deeper sleep, sometimes both dreaming REM sleep and the deeper so-called dreamless sleep. However, dreamless sleep is a misnomer. Our untrained minds are always generating images, sounds and feelings even in the deepest sleep states. After nearly twenty years of exploring my mind I can say with confidence that we are always dreaming, always aware. We usually do not consciously remember Delta experiences without training and effort.

Entrainment

One fairly simple and practical way we can change states of consciousness is through entrainment by experiencing rhythms related to these brainwave cycles. Some believe that staring at a candle flame or campfire produces an altered state of consciousness due to entrainment with the rhythmic flickering of the fire. Listening to tribal drumming can have the same effect.

Computer programs, biofeedback, audio recordings and other modern devices have been used for the last few decades to produce brainwave entrainment and they can be a great aid to state change. Of course they do not force you into altered states. They simply help you to find them more easily by providing a stimulation that your brain can start to imitate without even realizing.

One of the more common forms of these audio entrainment technologies is binaural beats which are rhythmic sounds created by slight frequency variations between the sound in the left and right ear. The rhythm is created by interference in the vibration caused by the different wavelengths. One of the more famous versions of this kind of technology is the "Hemi-Sync" technology created by the Monroe Institute. My own meditation recordings utilize a similar technology. Research has also shown that simple beats monaural beats or rhythmic sounds also work well in encouraging entrainment and altered states.

It should be mentioned however that no tool such as this can give you an experience of enlightenment, or even of true meditation, because meditation is not just about your nervous system, brain and brain waves. Meditation is about the intelligent use of different states of consciousness. No technology has produced meditation or enlightenment, and cannot do so, because these conditions are related to the skilful use of these brainwave conditions, not simply their presence.

As I said, all of the meditation recordings that I offer utilize embedded rhythmic sounds at various frequencies to help facilitate consciousness change. When conducting live classes and seminars I often use these sounds as an aid to participants. But I also share the consciousness focusing and transforming methods in this book at classes to really help people train and evolve their consciousness and awareness.

Simply Closing Your Eyes

Another excellent way to increase alpha brain waves is to just sit down and close your eyes. Research has shown definitively that in order to significantly increase alpha brain wave activity all that you need to do is close your eyes. So, if you just sit upright, close your eyes and rest for a few minutes you will find yourself feeling calm and centered quite quickly. Combining progressive relaxation with a few minutes with your eyes closed quickly delivers states of consciousness that relax the autonomic nervous system and provide most of the health benefits credited to meditation. So, if all you want is to relieve stress, just close your eyes and systematically relax your body. There are some simple instructions on this coming soon. If you add in some deep breathing to oxygenate your blood and encourage cell metabolism, nothing else is required to get 90% or more of the positive physiological effects of meditation. However, a bit more is required to get the long term evolutionary benefits.

The Thrupple of Attention

There are three main parts of your conscious inner experience of awareness and these are your vision, your hearing, and your feelings or sensations. All meditation explicitly uses one or more of these attention components as the tool for focus.

Our inner seeing sense is those images that we intentionally create such as visualizations and inner concentration objects, but also those memories, fantasies and imagery that come up without our intention. When we use an external object to focus upon visually, some of this noise is eliminated automatically, and this is one of the advantages of using an external object as a focal point for meditation.

Our inner hearing is any prayer or mantra you are repeating but also inner thinking, analyzing, planning, fantasizing or any other vocal or auditory experience that distracts from your meditation practice. One of the great values of repeating a word or sound over and over is that it makes it harder for inner verbalization to dominate.

Our inner feeling is both the emotions and kinesthetic sensations that you are creating intentionally as a meditation practice such as devotional enthusiasm or recollection of some experience but also the emotions that come up, such as fear, frustration, anxiety, etc., and also the positive and negative physical sensations that occur naturally such as postural discomfort or energy movements.

There are two other senses, smelling and tasting, and these play an important part in consciousness but not so much in inner consciousness. Smelling it is quite useful in memory and tasting is quite useful in arousing desires but neither of these are particularly what we're trying to do in cultivating focused meditation.

If you couple any two parts of consciousness together, let's say you combine hearing and seeing by repeating a sacred mantra while visualizing a divine image you have a much more stable basis of attention than focusing on just one element, just visualizing a divine image or just repeating a mantra. And if you combine all three parts: seeing, hearing and feeling, you form a very stable basis for your attention. Let's say you repeat a mantra while visualizing a divine image and pouring your heart out in loving devotion to the divine. This is a very full experience, and one that will make it quite a lot easier to maintain focus on a meditation object. All three parts of consciousness have one task. The mantra is the divine image in sound form, and the feeling connects all three.

I call this the "thrupple of attention," joining the three main components of your consciousness, seeing, hearing and feeling, into a single cohesive unit for focusing on the meditation object. So when you hear me mentioning the thrupple of attention throughout the rest of this book please know that I am referring to seeing hearing and feeling as a single unit, all connected in one task. And I want you to know that although I have given it a rather cheeky name, it is actually based upon quite traditional teaching sources in Yoga, Buddhism and Contemplative Christianity.

The most essential key to success in meditation is to take this thrupple of attention and give it a simple singular thing to do so that you may enter completely into the present moment. There is really no other way to be in the present moment other than to take your entire thrupple of attention and place it upon something. The more you can engage all three components in your practice, the more that the whole thrupple is involved, the more effective your practice will be.

If you are looking at a statue of the Dancing Shiva and chanting "AUM" but at the same time you are thinking about what you are going to do for the rest of the day once your practice is over, you are not engaging the full thrupple of your attention. Instead if you focus your entire visual awareness on that statue of Shiva, chant "AUM" and at the same time experience the great love and devotion you have toward Shiva as a distinct kinesthetic sense that is embodied in both the image of the statue and the sacred syllable "AUM" you are not going to be able to do anything else. This is engaging the thrupple of attention. All parts of your conscious awareness have a singular specific task in the present moment, and as long as the full thrupple is involved you are absorbed in reality.

However, it is highly important that this task is handled gently. Trying to force yourself to engage in this way aggressively is only going to result in rebellion from your consciousness. Instead, simply use the thrupple as your intended aim and happily return your attention to the thrupple whenever you notice all or part of your attention has drifted elsewhere. We will get back to this in more detail soon, but for now simply recognize that your attention needs to be maintained in the present, or returned to the present thrupple of attention as much as possible.

If you are not in this present moment giving your full attention to exactly what you are experiencing right now... you are either planning something for the future, thinking about something that happened earlier, or you are having some other sort of daydream, in any case you are not really experiencing reality in the present moment at all. You are not experiencing reality. Instead you are lost in things that are false, your inner fantasy analysis, your fears, your passions.

What's so magical about being in the present? That is where reality exists. Everything else is just a bunch of labels or things that simply don't exist at all. A huge amount of to our time is spent on fantasy about things that simply don't exist at all such as specific dates on the calendar or things to do with relationships and whether they are working, not working, or desired. We worry whether we are going to be on time. We worry about our possessions.

Every one of these things only exist in our minds. Dates on a calendar are completely made up and have been changed many times over the centuries. Relationships are commitments that we made up it in our heads that don't have any bearing on behavior or reality. Time is a completely made up concept that doesn't exist at all. Truly owning anything isn't possible since we ourselves are only a temporary phenomenon, and are at best borrowing from the universe on a very temporary basis.

Reality is just experiencing things as they are.

Clever people like to point out that Shiva, the "AUM" and the "devotion" described above do not necessarily represent present reality either. They are just constructs. This is true, however they are constructs created intentionally for the specific purpose of clarifying the awareness and stilling it within experience. They are like training wheels, which are abandoned when their purpose is spent. Many meditation practices utilize visualizations in one form or another as an entry point, but the real purpose of all practice is to still the mind and experience an open awareness of reality as it is. Most of the specific techniques we will discuss later focus only on reality as it is rather than utilizing those sorts of training wheels, although there are some advantages to them that we will discuss in the proper place.

When we take our attention, the thrupple of attention, and place it fully on something in our present awareness we come close to achieving a connection with reality. It is actually fairly rare in human consciousness to experience anything approximating reality.

When we can further free ourselves from the limiting descriptions of language we come ever closer to observing reality as it is. Reality without projections and fantasies is more ecstatically wonderful than imagination can allow. There is an amazing freedom that comes from releasing the need to control, understand or dominate our experience.

The actual process of meditating is extremely simple. All you need to do is take the thrupple of attention and aim it exclusively at something in awareness. Once no other internal representations are intruding on the process you are in present reality. You are experiencing reality as it is right now. When you cease to describe it and simply experience it you are in reality. This is the essence of meditation.

However as soon as you sit down and try to focus the thrupple of your attention upon some object you will notice something that may be a little disconcerting if you've never tried to meditate before.

What you will discover is the simple fact that you really don't have control over the contents of your mind at all. You intend to focus your attention and within moments unrelated thoughts have carried your attention far away from your meditation object. Unfocused and without clear intention, the thrupple of attention can be divided and think about multiple things at once. You may be aware of the sounds in the room around you while at the same time thinking about what you're going to do later today.

You don't have any control of it all but you do have the ability to train your mind. If you strain you will not get there. If you beat yourself up you will not get there.

The key is to make your focus loose and gentle at first, and to gently return your attention to the meditation object over and over again. Some people think that meditation involves intense and painful one-pointed focus. But this doesn't work, because you aren't in control. So, all that stressful, laser-like energy is no more effective than tranquil energy. Your mind wanders pretty quickly either way. But your mind likes pleasant experiences, so it is going to wander less if you approach things in a fun and relaxed way than if you approach with intensity or stress of any kind.

Meditation may at first seem like it might be boring, because you are just sitting there silently, apparently not doing much of anything. However, if you regularly engage the practices in this book, and perhaps use some of my related recordings, your meditation experience will quickly grow. It will become more interesting, you will be more engaged and have more fun. You will find that meditation will become something that you want to continue doing and you want to become good at doing.

Meditation is a lot like playing musical instruments or sports. The first time that you try to do it you discover that you're not very good at it and it may be noisy or even painful. But if you keep doing it you going to become a talented meditator in the same way that if you keep playing a musical instrument you will become an accomplished musician or keep playing a sport you will become a talented athlete.

Meditation has some important powers that neither music nor sports have. Meditation will deliver you calmness and peace of mind. Meditation will give you a greater sense of connection with the world around you. Meditation will help to make you a more authentic person, more truly representative of who you are.

While there are a variety of ways to approach meditation, there really only is one true technique, and that is to place your attention upon something and either to keep it there or else to keep returning it there as it drifts off in other directions. While some practices may seem to emphasize strongly focusing with intense one-pointed powerful intention, while others ask you to hold on loosely, allowing consciousness to quiet passively, this is misleading. While these two seem distinct, they have the same purpose which is to center the attention on some object. They are really the same instruction. If your "intense" focus is straining, struggling, sweating and beating yourself up for your shifting attention, it is not in fact leading toward anything but suffering and tension. The intensity of your will related to meditation needs to simply be a strong commitment to relaxed focus.

Lucid vs. Sluggish Relaxation

Relaxation is essential to meditation. However, relaxing too much or the wrong way is a hazard, especially once you are more familiar with the process and you start to relax easily. It is even possible to fall completely asleep sitting completely bolt upright. I have heard a lot of snoring around me on longer meditation retreats, and I have even awoken myself with a snore on more than one occasion. But relaxation is still essential to the process of meditation.

Many people are afraid to relax and let their mind become loose and open. There is very little understanding of states of consciousness in our culture. Words like hypnosis, trance, altered states and so on conjure up fantasy images of people losing control of themselves in the hands of unscrupulous charlatans. However, the ability of people to manipulate the minds of others has very little to do with any particular state of consciousness, but rather with using manipulative behaviors. You should feel very comfortable allowing yourself to relax. It is a healing state.

Some people resist the idea of relaxing because they feel it is a form of laziness or an attempt to escape from reality. However, relaxation is one of the most important tools we have in meditation practice. Some people believe relaxation is not a part of meditation because you must remain vigilant about focusing on your meditation object. While this focus is important, relaxation can be a powerful ally in doing just that.

The more relaxed you are, the more you are not distracted by verbal thought, conceptualizations about the past and future, bodily sensations or anything else. But it is far easier to relax and zone out than to relax in a way that maintains a lucid awareness. When I first started meditating I really wanted to get out of my head and so I sought states in which my consciousness was basically disappearing. I was getting so out of it that I was fading out into a pleasant, grey, emptiness. This kind of sluggish relaxed state can be very pleasant and is pretty easily attained. However it doesn't really accomplish anything more than offering an escape. Like a drug, this kind of state can be enjoyable, but doesn't lead anywhere.

It was much later before I realized that in fact it is just a slightly different state that we are seeking. We can and should relax as deeply as possible, however at the same time we must keep the mind clear and lucid. Meditation is not a state of relaxed fuzziness, but a state of relaxed attention. This is somewhat easier said than done but it is not truly all that hard. It is simply a matter of training your mind to notice a few key indicators.

If you are finding your mind thinking too much, constantly returning to planning, analyzing or narrating your experience, relaxing more will take care of this. If you are finding yourself agitated or bored with your meditation, relaxing more deeply will help you to feel happier and more tranquil in your practice. It will make your practice feel better.

You must simply balance relaxation with attentiveness. If you notice that your thinking process is impaired, such as you are forgetting what you are doing, then you have gone too far toward relaxation. If you notice a strong sense of sleepiness or dullness, you have become too relaxed. If your visual awareness seems weakened, a fuzziness around the periphery, or if you feel a bodily sense of falling, you are becoming too relaxed.

The remedy is to take a greater interest in the meditation object with the thrupple of attention. It may also be useful to take a few deeper breaths, or a few faster breaths if you are already breathing deeply. You can even adjust your posture slightly if you are really nodding off.

What you want to do is bring your attention to bear upon the meditation object in a completely focused way that at the same time remains calm and unattached. You can softly focus on your attention upon the object with the thrupple of attention. Just allow yourself to gently see, hear and feel, without letting go but without holding on too tightly.

Attentional Reward vs. Distraction Punishment

Meditation is extremely simple to do. All you need to do is sit there and be quietly aware of what is, without becoming lost in thoughts about the past or the future, or even about what the present is about. The problem is that your mind is not accustomed this activity and as soon as you set the intention to "sit there" your mind begins to look for other things to do.

There is an important key to meditation that is often mentioned, but its importance is often overlooked. See, you can't actually consciously force yourself to "do meditation" for any length of time, because you are not actually in control of your consciousness. You are really just along for the ride. Awareness pops up in many different ways over and over again, but it also tends to fade or shift elsewhere.

So, it becomes necessary to have some sort of way to get all of the competing pieces of consciousness working together if we are going to meditate. Otherwise meditation sessions become daydream sessions.

When you get angry at yourself for getting distracted, it serves really no point whatsoever, because "you" aren't getting distracted. It is any one of many other components of your consciousness that is causing and getting distracted. If you were in control, you would do the practice perfectly. Right? All that getting agitated by distraction does is make the various components of your consciousness less likely to notice distraction. Why would you want that unpleasant experience? Instead your mind will just stay distracted because then there is no problem. If you get mad at yourself you will train yourself to avoid the pain by never noticing that you are distracted.

If on the other hand, when you notice that you are distracted you feel good that you noticed it, you will find yourself noticing it more and more, and staying on task more and more until very quickly you find yourself totally absorbed.

At first, your attention will flag and stray pretty regularly. Just return it to the task at hand when you notice that you have drifted. Make sure that you take a moment to feel good for noticing that you have wandered, rather than feeling bad for mind wandering. It is possible to get distracted for long periods. Your goal is to shorten these and eventually to be able to focus with unbroken attention. The only way to train your mind is to reward the noticing. Rewarding the noticing makes your awareness recognize that the goal is concentration. Punishing the wandering is only going to make your mind wander more because until you notice it the wandering goes unpunished and so your awareness will keep wandering and never let you notice to avoid punishment. This has been demonstrated in studies.

You are going to be holding several things in attention at once, and it is one of these that has been replaced by the distraction. So, after congratulating yourself for noticing the distraction, determine which part of the thrupple of attention got replaced by the distraction, and then calmly reengage with the whole thrupple.

It may take several weeks of practice for there to be extended periods where your consciousness stays on task . Do not let yourself get discouraged as this is another form of punishment and will negatively affect your commitment to practice. Instead, utilize the stages of practice discussed later to create a goal for your practice that is reasonable. In other words, at level one, just set a goal to be staying focused 50% of the time. Once you achieve this regularly, move you goal to level two, and so on. Very soon you will find yourself experiencing the wonderful levels of bliss that accompany full meditative absorption.

Foveal vs. Peripheral Awareness

Foveal vision is the focus of attention at the center of the lens of your eye, and tends to be clear and sharp. On the other hand peripheral awareness is vision at the outer edges of sight. These two components of vision are intimately related with the conscious mind and the unconscious components of your biology. In fact, this section could also be called Consciousness vs. Unconsciousness. One of the most valuable ways that you can increase your deepest awareness is to become aware of the foveal and peripheral in your visual perception right now, and to allow your awareness to gently encompass both. Do the same with the sensations in your body until you are aware of your whole body as a field of sensation. Do the same with your inner verbalizations by ceasing to be caught up in identifying with thoughts, but instead recognizing where the various thoughts and related imagery are coming from. This is the thrupple of attention in **open awareness**. This is what meditation is designed to facilitate.

Our conscious mind is only that portion of awareness that is focused upon anything at the moment. Every other part of experience is in the greater awareness of our consciousness but outside of our present focus. Meditation offers us an opportunity to become more attuned to more and more of this experience in our bodies, in our feelings and sensations, in the conscious thoughts that describe our experience and the unconscious patterns of thought and belief that define the limits of our being.

Meditation offers a conduit between our conscious and unconscious through three main bridges. The first and easiest bridge is our breath. Our breath is run effortlessly by our unconscious nervous system, but we can easily take control of the process, deepen it, suspend it, or make it very rapid. Then, as soon as we stop playing in this way, our unconscious takes back the reins and returns our breathing to the rhythm most appropriate for our bodily needs. Meditation techniques that focus on the breath are very common because of this, and their great power lies in large part in this connection between the conscious and unconscious.

The second bridge is through sensation. As I mentioned previously, we edit out a large percentage of the sensory information we are taking in until it is necessary and sometimes not even then. Have you ever been sitting for a long period concentrating on something only to discover your legs have fallen asleep? The sensation was always there but we didn't pay attention. Further, we can create sensations and even emotions through using our consciousness. Can you think of what it is like to be happy? Where do you feel the pleasant sensations of happiness in your body? Allow yourself to feel those sensations in those places right now.

The third bridge is thought. This includes both verbalization and inner imagery. While we frequently feel we are in control of this verbalization, a few minutes trying to silence the mind quickly demonstrates how much is going on that we are not controlling or even instigating. As we examine the mind more carefully it becomes clear that there are whole areas of thought that influence our actions that we barely become cognizant of consciously.

So, utilizing the various meditation vehicles through the thrupple of attention allows us to become more presently aware of all of these components in our consciousness. This eventually allows us to dispense with many of the less positive components and to more vividly experience those that are skilful and serene.

Habituation vs. Seeking Novelty

One of the most common and tricky challenges facing every meditator is that after a certain number of sitting sessions the whole process becomes well known and so there is a strong tendency for the mind to turn it into a habit. The problem with this is that your mind will then start trying to do other things "while meditating" such as planning your day or musing on some philosophical idea. It is even possible to hold onto the meditation object at least partially and engage in these sorts of thoughts. This, of course, eventually leads us to no longer meditating at all.

The best way to manage this is to very strongly consider the practice of meditation to be something that is constantly developing, unfolding and emerging, and an activity which you need to treat as almost a sort of treasure hunt. If you are panning for gold you are going to look at every grain of sand quite carefully so that you do not miss out on that elusive chunk of ore. Meditation needs to be approached with a similar attention to detail.

Instead of a lump of metal, you are seeking a complete and real perception of your meditative object that will allow you to see truly experience the deepest truths of reality. Make sure that you keep your practice fresh by really focusing as vividly as possible on the colors, feelings, energies and process every time, and making it your intention to do it more and more deeply and effectively each time. This is why we take a moment at the beginning of each practice to be very conscious about our purpose so that we can see each sitting as the fresh opportunity for transformation that it truly is.

Beliefs, Opinions and Preferences

These have nothing to do with the practice or experience of meditation, and actually form some of the most pervasive challenges to practice as you are sitting, but also between practices when you are deciding how to spend your time. The more you can establish an open and tranquil approach to meditation without any preconceived expectations or other mental baggage, the quicker you will be able to become fully absorbed in your practice.

At first, the mental challenges will center around whether the practice is worthwhile, whether you are doing it right, or whether you are doing the right practice for you. Over time you will start to add desires to get your friends and family to start meditating, how meditation fits with whatever religious inclinations and traditions you maintain, and other social aspects. Eventually you will add various theories, philosophical notions, and comparative spiritual models to your thinking. All of these matters are distractions from your meditation practice and the more you can avoid thinking about this sort of stuff the better off you will be in your journey.

Beliefs in general are just fantasies about things we don't know to be true. Otherwise it is not a belief, it is a knowing. Placing a lot of importance upon beliefs takes you further from reality, not closer. Beliefs tend to lead toward animosity against people who think differently and ultimately toward the dark path of religious fundamentalism. For the most part, beliefs are bad for your spiritual development. They are just labels and thoughts, meaningless encumbrances.

The answers to life's great questions are not going to be found in your thoughts and fantasies. The answers will be found when you let go of them.

Breathing, Relaxation and Your Body

I am now going to reveal a little secret. I've actually already mentioned it, but now I am going to be very explicit. Most of the health benefits credited to meditation can be accomplished with no skill whatsoever simply engaging deep breathing and/or progressive relaxation. Not coincidentally, a lot of meditation techniques center around breath and relaxation. Meditation itself is not about breath or relaxation, it is about gently focused awareness. But breath and relaxation are the two most powerful tools you have to develop this focused awareness. As previously mentioned, breath is a powerful bridge between our various levels of consciousness, and it is also a facilitator of the parasympathetic nervous system response.

Take a Deep Breath

Ten to twenty slow and deep breaths can significantly lower heart rate, blood pressure and produce feelings of comfort and peace that are completely undeniable. Go ahead and give it a try. Count on your fingers and take ten or more very deep breaths. Notice how you feel afterwards. Go ahead, I'll wait.

Feels pretty good, right? Keep doing it for fifteen to twenty minutes and you will feel amazing.

Breathing has a truly profound effect on our consciousness. Deep breathing relaxes us very quickly. If we breathe rapidly and deeply enough we can change our consciousness in almost psychedelic ways. Breathing affects our cellular metabolism increasing our health in numerous ways. In the pranayama practices that follow in a later section, you will learn to utilize the transformative effects of powerful breathwork in ways that increase your personal energy and also allow you greater presence for deeply examining awareness with the thrupple of attention.

Relaxation

Bodily relaxation plays an incredibly important part in our consciousness development as well as in our health and in our well being but it is viewed a little strangely by a lot of society. Relaxation can seem less interesting than various other kinds of entertainment. Taking time to relax can also be considered laziness. Even among spiritual people relaxation is sometimes viewed as a lazy approach to spirituality that only leads to vague states of reverie and zoning out. This largely comes from a view towards spirituality that is largely punitive in that people believe that by doing difficult or challenging things they are going to somehow make up for bad things they did in the past. This is an almost universal phenomenon. We see this in ascetic communities in India where severe physical postures are endured for long periods of time in order to burn off bad karma. Punishing periods of fasting or exposure to the elements are also used. Practices of self flagellation and fasting are popular amongst many Christian spiritual seekers for very similar reasons other than the replacement of the word "sin" for the word "karma."

To people who have been trained to see such extreme behaviors as required for spiritual development, the idea that you could get spiritual benefit from deep relaxation might seem pretty unbelievable. For such, sitting in an uncomfortable difficult posture for hours while staring intently at the sun might seem like a more profitable method of meditation.

But the physical health benefits of regular relaxation are completely undeniable, and are in fact the most well researched cause of the beneficial effects of meditation. Popular meditation courses such as

Transcendental Meditation or Mindfulness Based Stress Reduction are really based in large part upon relaxation, though some of their practitioners might disagree. But if you do not relax as you are repeating the mantra or while being mindful of breathing, you are not going to be doing either very effectively. Deep mental and physical relaxation is a key component to both practices.

One of the great effects of meditation is the moving away from the fight or flight mechanism toward the rest and digest state. The direct action of a good meditation practice on the nervous system is that it activates the parasympathetic nervous system to relax your body and consciousness completely. But a guided progressive relaxation of your whole body or even simply deep breathing has exactly the same effect on the nervous system as meditation so if you are simply looking for the relaxing sedative effect of meditation you don't need to bother with any other tools in this book aside from simply deep breathing and learning to relax your muscles. There is a lot of research on relaxation and deep breathing both of which have been shown to have powerful effects upon the parasympathetic system.

Truthfully however, when you do deep breathing or relaxation you will feel really good for a while but it doesn't last forever. Slowly, as you go about your day-to-day life after you're done with your progressive relaxation or deep breathing, the nervous system begins to shift back to its normal patterns. At first you will feel untouchable. Your children will scream. You'll find out that a bill is late and something's being shut off. None of it will affect you in slightest, and you will say, "Oh my goodness I'm enlightened now."

But after a while the effects of this will wear off and you will start feeling angered and upset once again. This can really be equally true of all meditation, including Mindfulness and Transcendental Meditation. When you conclude your session you feel really nice. You feel great but it doesn't last forever. Eventually the effects wear off. It is a temporary fix. It is like putting a pain killing compound on a thorn that's stuck into the side of your leg. You put the pain killer on it stops killing the pain for a while but, as long as the thorn is still there, there can be no permanent relief.

The only permanent relief comes by removing the thorn. The thorn in our consciousness is the persistent ego perception that there is an individual "I" that is fragile, important and must be hidden from the world. The only way to permanently remove the thorn of ego is to really change our consciousness.

Meditation eventually can do this basically automatically by allowing you to more and more clearly see what reality really is and what reality isn't. Simply by sitting on your meditation seat and bringing the thrupple of attention more and more to bear upon a meditation object you will eventually experience things as they are without the interruption of your thoughts and ideas. Once you stabilize this you are enlightened. True enlightenment still contains all possible behaviors but frees awareness from being compelled by them. To the extent you are compelled by anything or afraid of anything you are not enlightened. To the extent that you can be content and happy under any circumstances, free from judgment, worry, hate or desire, you are enlightened.

Stumbling Blocks in Meditation Practice

Most spiritual meditation instructions begin with an extensive requirement for purification, morally and ethically, before commencing your meditation practices. In the *Yoga Sutras* of Patanjali, the first steps preliminary to meditation are called *yama* and *niyama*. These are the "thou shalts" and "thou shalt nots" of *Astanga* Yoga. They consist of harmlessness, truthfulness, non-stealing, chastity, non-greed, purity, contentment, austerity, study and surrender to the divine. These are quite similar in almost every particular to the ten commandments of the Semitic Religions. Christian Mystics often add a requirement to be "confessed" and to have recently received the "sacrament of communion." Buddhism has a list of five moral precepts for lay practitioners that consists of abstaining from taking life, stealing, sexual misconduct, lying, or taking intoxicants. The list of precepts for Buddhist monks and nuns can involve hundreds of rules, depending upon the specific sect we are talking about.

All of these may seem like rather arbitrary religious sentiments that have little or nothing to do with improving our focused awareness or relaxation, and so perhaps irrelevant to meditation. Moral purification doesn't seem to have much to do with any of the rest of what we have been talking about so far in our practical approach to meditation. However, if you look at all of the suggested behaviors, they are the natural behaviors of an enlightened being, freed from ego. They are the way we would all act if we weren't caught up in selfish dramas, desires and fears.

These items do also in fact have quite an impact on our practice, in utterly practical, non-spiritual, non-moralistic terms. You see, if your life is filled with drama from all your boozing, high seas piracy and sexual misadventures when you sit down to meditate you are going to find your mind is quite agitated, all the time. If after some time you finally get relaxed enough to focus, thoughts about your past or future adventures are going to continuously pop in to plague you because they have made a big impression upon your consciousness. And not just from being a pirate! Everything that you do leaves an impression in consciousness and as you are trying to concentrate, you are going to get disturbed by your day's activities over and over.

So, the simpler you make your life, the easier it is going to be to get into a relaxed and concentrated state, and to stay there. So, adopting some form of the above injunctions is an entirely practical instruction that has nothing to do with placating deities or invisible spirits. It has to do with improving your ability to practice easily.

Also, at the end of every meditation practice you are going to feel very relaxed, happy and blissful. When your life is very chaotic, filled with drama, heavy emotion and passionate adventures, you are going to find the "afterglow" of meditation is very short-lived, whereas if you are living a tranquil stress-free life, you feel as if you are walking on air for the whole day after an extended meditation session. You will particularly notice this if you ever have the opportunity for an extended meditation retreat. While you are on retreat you may feel enlightened, but once you get home and you discover your kids smashed the living room television during the kegger they threw in your absence, suddenly that enlightenment can turn into rage pretty fast.

Another hidden benefit of avoiding a lot of sensory stimulation in your life is that the rewards of meditation are actually far more wonderful than the material benefits of a decadent life. But they are far more subtle, so they are not as easily noticed if you are overly engaged in material pleasures. In the same way that you are going to miss out on the delicate flavors of a gourmet meal by dumping ketchup all over your plate, you will miss out on the subtle pleasures of meditative bliss if your mind is fixated on sex, drugs and rock'n'roll.

However, this is better experienced than discussed. I think t' that you should not meditate until you are pure is p' backwards. If I tell you to stop drinking wine meditate more effectively that is probably goin' to take something away from you and w' helping you toward enlightenment, this Suffering is never something you should c yourself carefully and engaging in your looking at what is coming up as a distraction most often, and attempting to simplify your life in a more practical way as it becomes obvious what things are making it harder to practice and what behaviors outside of practice help you maintain your happiness and which ones do not. Then you will naturally move in the direction that is best for you, and when you find yourself following all the injunctions above and more it will be because they are a natural expression of your being rather than something you are trying to force on yourself.

The Five Hindrances

In Buddhist meditation there is a specific list of five experiences in awareness that block our ability to enter meditative absorption. They are called the five hindrances to meditation. When our mind is engaged in these, we are not absorbed, when it is free from these, we are absorbed in meditation. These hindrances are:

- Sensory desires
- Ill-will
- Sloth and torpor
- Worry and restlessness
- Doubt

The meditation practices will naturally remove you from these hindrances temporarily, but when we return to normal life we return to these hindrances. Only once we have begun to adopt the purifications and live a more simple life can we begin to see these hindrances disappear on a more permanent basis. In each meditation practice the hindrances disappear temporarily slowly after we engage our practice method meticulously for an extended period of time. They will only reemerge later, after we discontinue our meditation practice. As our practice ripens they take longer and longer to reemerge.

Early Christian mystics had a very similar list of mental hindrances, eight in number, which they associated with the subtle attacks and temptations of demons on the consciousness of the monk. These were thoughts related to:

- Gluttony
- Fornication
- Avarice
- Anger
- Sadness
- Restlessness
- Vainglory
- Pride

This list was later edited and transformed into the "seven deadly sins," and applied more generally to the population and their behaviors, but the original conception related to the distractions and temptations distinctive to the life of an ascetic monk. As you can see, although the second list is slightly longer, it covers exactly the same material. These are all the exact thoughts and feelings that will distract a monk from meditation, and will distract you from your meditation practice too. So, the more we can simplify our lives the easier it will be to experience the benefits of meditation over the long term.

Stumbling Blocks in Meditation Practice

Most spiritual meditation instructions begin with an extensive requirement for purification, morally and ethically, before commencing your meditation practices. In the *Yoga Sutras* of Patanjali, the first steps preliminary to meditation are called *yama* and *niyama*. These are the "thou shalts" and "thou shalt nots" of *Astanga* Yoga. They consist of harmlessness, truthfulness, non-stealing, chastity, non-greed, purity, contentment, austerity, study and surrender to the divine. These are quite similar in almost every particular to the ten commandments of the Semitic Religions. Christian Mystics often add a requirement to be "confessed" and to have recently received the "sacrament of communion." Buddhism has a list of five moral precepts for lay practitioners that consists of abstaining from taking life, stealing, sexual misconduct, lying, or taking intoxicants. The list of precepts for Buddhist monks and nuns can involve hundreds of rules, depending upon the specific sect we are talking about.

All of these may seem like rather arbitrary religious sentiments that have little or nothing to do with improving our focused awareness or relaxation, and so perhaps irrelevant to meditation. Moral purification doesn't seem to have much to do with any of the rest of what we have been talking about so far in our practical approach to meditation. However, if you look at all of the suggested behaviors, they are the natural behaviors of an enlightened being, freed from ego. They are the way we would all act if we weren't caught up in selfish dramas, desires and fears.

These items do also in fact have quite an impact on our practice, in utterly practical, non-spiritual, non-moralistic terms. You see, if your life is filled with drama from all your boozing, high seas piracy and sexual misadventures when you sit down to meditate you are going to find your mind is quite agitated, all the time. If after some time you finally get relaxed enough to focus, thoughts about your past or future adventures are going to continuously pop in to plague you because they have made a big impression upon your consciousness. And not just from being a pirate! Everything that you do leaves an impression in consciousness and as you are trying to concentrate, you are going to get disturbed by your day's activities over and over.

So, the simpler you make your life, the easier it is going to be to get into a relaxed and concentrated state, and to stay there. So, adopting some form of the above injunctions is an entirely practical instruction that has nothing to do with placating deities or invisible spirits. It has to do with improving your ability to practice easily.

Also, at the end of every meditation practice you are going to feel very relaxed, happy and blissful. When your life is very chaotic, filled with drama, heavy emotion and passionate adventures, you are going to find the "afterglow" of meditation is very short-lived, whereas if you are living a tranquil stress-free life, you feel as if you are walking on air for the whole day after an extended meditation session. You will particularly notice this if you ever have the opportunity for an extended meditation retreat. While you are on retreat you may feel enlightened, but once you get home and you discover your kids smashed the living room television during the kegger they threw in your absence, suddenly that enlightenment can turn into rage pretty fast.

Another hidden benefit of avoiding a lot of sensory stimulation in your life is that the rewards of meditation are actually far more wonderful than the material benefits of a decadent life. But they are far more subtle, so they are not as easily noticed if you are overly engaged in material pleasures. In the same way that you are going to miss out on the delicate flavors of a gourmet meal by dumping ketchup all over your plate, you will miss out on the subtle pleasures of meditative bliss if your mind is fixated on sex, drugs and rock'n'roll.

However, this is better experienced than discussed. I think the injunction that you should not meditate until you are pure is putting things a bit backwards. If I tell you to stop drinking wine at night so you can meditate more effectively that is probably going to feel like I am wanting to take something away from you and will cause suffering. Instead of helping you toward enlightenment, this will push you further from it. Suffering is never something you should do. I would suggest observing yourself carefully and engaging in your meditation practice, slowly

Approaching Meditation Skillfully

We have already gone over several strategies that will help you quickly grow into a skilful and enlightened meditator. When you apply these factors to your practice you will find yourself growing almost immediately. In a nutshell, these factors are focusing the full thrupple of attention, rewarding your awareness, relaxing in a lucid manner, opening to the unconscious, and always seeking to keep the practice fresh and new.

The Buddhists define seven factors of enlightened awareness. In contrast to their five mental conditions that block our access to meditative absorption, there are seven mental conditions that encourage an enlightened state. These are:

- Mindfulness
- Investigation
- Energy
- Joy
- Tranquility
- Concentration
- Equanimity

The twentieth sutra of the first chapter of the *Yoga Sutras* contains a similar list of factors:

- Certainty
- Energy
- Mindfulness
- Concentration
- Wisdom

If you look carefully, you can see that my factors and the Buddhist and Yogic factors are not all that different.

When these factors are all present, we are fully engaged in our practice, and in enlightened awareness. When any are missing, we are requiring balance of one sort or another. Mindfulness is the factor that has received the most attention in Western science based studies of meditation, and is considered to be a requisite for all the rest. It is the state of present awareness of what is going on. If you are not present, you cannot do your meditation practice at all. You will just be sitting there daydreaming about the past or the future.

The next six can be divided into two basic groups, those that increase tranquility, and those that energize. A background awareness of these can be quite useful when you are trying to balance between getting sleepy in meditation, and being overly agitated.

When you are getting sleepy, you can intentionally become more interested in and curious about your meditation object, utilizing the enlightenment factor of investigation. Or you can put more intention into your practice, using the energy enlightenment factor. Or you can become more joyful about your practice.

When you are feeling anxious, agitated or irritable, you can intentionally relax your body more deeply using the tranquility factor. You can also rest your attention with greater stillness upon the object, or intentionally let go of all cares in general, instead simply being with the object equanimously.

This is how these enlightenment factors can be practical tools in your meditation practice.

The Five Basic Levels of Meditative Skill

At first when you begin your meditation practice you are not going to be very good at it. Your mind is going to wander constantly and you are going to wonder if meditation is even a real possibility, or if your mind is just too wild to ever get under control. Luckily, you are going to make progress, and if you carefully observe, you will see yourself improving regularly. Over the centuries there have been numerous maps of progress proposed by various religions and sects. Some of them are incredibly detailed and elaborate. However, for our purposes, we will define five basic stages. This is enough for us to realistically gauge progress in a general way that is extremely clear and lacks ambiguity.

We are not going to spend a great deal of time on these but I want you to be aware that there is a simple progression of skill that you can observe happening within yourself as you start to meditate consistently. Each of these stages will naturally develop in sequence if you follow the simple instructions throughout this book.

Learning – Level One

At the first stage of meditation practice, you are just learning a technique. You will quickly find that almost as soon as you focus your attention on the meditation object your mind goes off to something else. The meditation object comes and goes frequently. Whole mediation sessions can come and go almost totally engaged in daydreaming or zoning out.

Goal: establishing a regular daily practice and increasing your attention to more than 50% of the time on the meditation object.

Enemies: distraction, daydreaming, planning, etc.

Developing – Level Two

You will have reached this level when the meditation object stays in awareness more than 50% of the time. Distractions will still be frequent, but you hold onto the object through them at least half the time.

Goal: 100% sustained awareness of the object even through distraction.

Enemies: mind wandering, restlessness

Fixating – Level Three

At this level you will be able to sustain your awareness of the object throughout your session, even if distractions come up. Your mind may still maintain some turbulence here and there, but most of your attention is occupied keeping the object in awareness.

Goal: Centered absorption in the object that is not affected by distraction. Thoughts about the object may still come up, as well as occasional distractions, but your focus is sustained on the object.

Enemies: sluggishness, sleepiness, dullness

Absorbing – Level Four

At this stage you enter into complete fixation on the object. At first this will require effort, but will become automatic as you continue to engage with the practice over time.

Goal: Effortless absorption

Enemies: Dryness, frustration, fear

Mastering – Level Five

At this level focusing is effortless. Your mind takes hold of the meditation object automatically and your consciousness melts into a completely present and centered focus.

Goal: mastering individual types of jhana or samadhi

Enemies: various distracting energy phenomena

These five simple stages take us from non-meditator to absorption in jhana or samadhi.

Learning	-	easily distracted
Developing	-	sometimes distracted
Fixating	-	getting focused
Absorbing	-	intently focused
Mastering	-	effortless focus

The Four Stages of Absorption

As you progress in your practice, you are going to begin experiencing states that are extremely blissful and ecstatic. These states are the result of being free from the five hindrances previously described while being deeply engrossed in your practice. There are a number of different maps for these experiences, and I want to briefly explore them before moving to the practical steps before us.

Once you are no longer experiencing any pull from distractions of any kind, physical, emotional, or mental you are going to find yourself slipping into various levels of absorption into the object of contemplation. These experiences are accompanied by various ecstasies, seeing lights, colors, heavenly sounds and other energy phenomena. Buddhists call these the four Jhanas. There is some disagreement about the exact meaning of these jhanas, so I will just share what is agreed upon.

- First Jhana - occurs when consciousness is secluded from the five hindrances. It is defined by an experience of rapture and pleasure. There is still discursive thought present at least occasionally
- Second Jhana - there is still rapture and pleasure, but discursive thought is no longer present
- Third Jhana - there is still pleasure, but rapture has ceased and is replaced by equanimity
- Fourth Jhana - only equanimity remains

The seclusion from the five hindrances described above is a natural conclusion of the deeply relaxed and focused state produced by the meditation techniques that will follow in the next sections.

While a similar set of factors can be found in his sutras, Pantanjali's yoga outlines a slightly different four phase description of the stages of concentration, contained within its eight limbs or steps. Interestingly the third entry Dhyana is the Sanskrit linguistic cognate of the Pali word Jhana above.

- Pratyahara – The senses are withdrawn from other external objects to be focused on the meditation object
- Dharana – The state of intense focus on the meditation object
- Dhyana – The state of absorption in the meditation object
- Samadhi – The state of unification with the meditation object

It is also interesting to note that the fourth stage of each of the above models is where both traditions state the practitioner starts to develop paranormal abilities such as telepathy and psychokinesis.

There is a further four stage refinement of concentration called samapatti which is described in the *Yoga Sutras*, based upon the meditation object itself. Unification is divided up into mentally supported (with a mantra or similar) concentration or unsupported, on material (gross) or formless (subtle) objects. In this case a formless object is something like "the divine" as a pure concept. Unsupported concentration on a formless object is of course considered the most advanced.

- Savitarka – concentration on gross objects with words
- Savichara – concentration on subtle objects with words
- Nirvitarka – concentration on gross objects without words
- Nirvichara – concentration on subtle objects without words

Notice that these yogic models are about the functional behaviors while the Buddhist model is more about the internal experience of the practitioner which makes it somewhat easier to understand the Buddhist model even if the Yogic model may be more complete in some ways.

In contemplative Christianity there are usually considered to be three much simpler stages in the process of becoming enlightened.

- Katharsis – purification of the soul
- Theoria – divine illumination of the soul
- Theosis – becoming one with God

This model could be valuable for some practitioners to see. The first stage is about dropping the sensual desires and egoic consciousness in general. The second stage is about opening to the grace of direct experience of the divine and the third is complete absorption in that grace.

All of these differing models can be enlightening, but they can also become confusing or allow us to engage in fantasies of various kinds. Their real value is in the simple awareness that there is in fact a growth process underway and that if we just continue to do what we are doing we will experience ever growing transformation and peace.

PART 2 – MEDITATION TOOLS AND PARTS

While the practice of meditation can be as simple as just sitting down and concentrating on an object of your choice for a prescribed period of time, most people find this to be both dry and difficult, because the mind starts out quite agitated and thoughts about other matters or what we are going to do after the practice tend to dominate the practice for a considerable time. By easing into the practice with a few preliminaries, you can focus more easily and devote more of your practice period to growth rather than simply to struggling with the process. Mind you, there will still be times in which you struggle, but these additional supports will help to keep you along the path toward success.

I have developed a simple eight step process that you can engage quite easily each time you sit down to practice.

1. POSTURE – establishing an upright seated position in which are comfortable but won't fall asleep
2. RECOLLECTION OF INTENT - establishing a clear unselfish enlightened goal and intention for the meditation
3. BREATHING – a few minutes of simple deep breathing to shift awareness
4. RELAXING - relaxing as deeply as possible to release any stress or hindrance
5. THE CENTRAL PRACTICE – a prescribed time focusing on the meditation object with the thrupple of attention
6. ELEVATING EMOTIONS – establishing positive uplifted emotional states
7. FUTURE PACING - setting the clear intent to experience this calm loving energy more in our future
8. SHARING BENEFITS - freely sharing the benefits of the practice with everyone we care about

This framework around the basic practice is based upon both mediation traditions and a massive amount of clinical and personal research that shows these particular exercises add greatly to the rapid success of meditative practice. The preliminary awareness exercises prepare your consciousness for transformation and set your state with calming breaths and relaxation. Then in this relaxed and focused state you will engage your meditation practice for fifteen minutes to an hour.

After the central practice you will conclude with elevating your emotional state, future pacing, and sharing the benefits creating a kind attitude toward everyone. This process creates very positive neuro-associations with the practice and creates a greater sense of connection with your environment. Put together, this eight-step process makes every session an opportunity for significant personal growth on multiple levels while the attention is being trained to engage more fully. There is no such thing as a "bad session" with this system, because you are always going to be experiencing something positive.

Many spiritual or religious meditation forms utilize ritual of various kinds as a preliminary to meditation. Such rituals allow for a transition from the mundane secular world, opening the door to a more spiritual realm. The simple eight part formula above allows us to engage with the best aspects of ritualized behavior, the conditioned response for transition to practice, without any inherent spiritual baggage. It is also recommended that you meditate in the same place regularly as it will amplify this effect.

I want to mention again that you can jump into this very easily by utilizing my audio recordings which guide you through all of the steps we will go over in the rest of the book in a simple and easy way. They also contain embedded binaural sounds that encourage brainwave state change which also provides a shield from distracting noise in the environment. I am the father of three children and sometimes those background binaural sounds are very necessary to allow me to engage in my own practice. We will now go over each of these parts in detail.

The Preliminary Stretch

Before getting started on your daily meditation practice, I highly recommend taking a few minutes to stretch and get your body loosened before getting seated as it really will make sitting more comfortable and allow your nervous system to react more favorably to the experience. Here is an outline of my usual stretching routine.

You may notice that while all of these practices are found within modern Yoga classes, it does not contain a number of the more popular poses such as "Downward Dog," or the "Tree Pose." That is because the poses selected here are for the specific purpose of preparing the body for seated meditation. You could also do a full postural Yoga routine before meditating, but that is not necessary. These simple stretches open your hips, stretch your spine, and generally prepare your body for sitting for an extended period quite well. Obviously, do the sequence twice, focusing on both your right and left side.

- UTTANASANA - Forward bend
- BHUJANGASANA - Cobra stretch
- UTTHAN PRISTHASANA - Runner's lunge
- KAPOTASANA - Pigeon pose
- AGNISTAMBHASANA - Double pigeon
- PADMASANA - Full Lotus or Half lotus
- ARDHA MATSYENDRASANA - Seated Spinal Twist
- MAHAMUDRA - Seated forward bend with one legged tucked under groin
- PASCHIMOTTANASANA - Seated forward bend

Detailed instructions on these fairly simple stretches can be found all over the Internet but would take up too much space here.

I generally take five very deep breaths in each of these positions. This engages the relaxation response as well as keeping me from shortening some of the more challenging stretches.

You can also conduct these stretches again after sitting practice.

Posture

Your sitting posture is of such great importance to your success in meditation that I am dedicating a whole step in the process to its establishment. Many modern meditation instructors just advise you to sit in a "comfortable upright posture," and while this is the right instruction, it is very oversimplified. If you are sitting wrong, your body is going to bother you throughout your practice with aches in your back, neck, shoulders or legs. If you sit correctly, you will soon discover that you can sit almost indefinitely with no greater difficulty than perhaps your legs getting a bit tingly.

At my first long meditation retreat I spent the second through the sixth days in a constant state of agony, until I figured out on my own how to sit correctly. However, the process is well known among the Yogis of Tibet, India and Japan. Had my instructor simply given me the correct method it would have been a lot easier to succeed in that retreat! But again, there seems to be a contingent in the spiritual community that believes physical pain and suffering belong in the path to awakening. I remember going to a Sikh Kundalini Yoga class one time and they had us hold out arms out at a forty five degree angle for five minutes straight or more. When we put our arms down there was a powerful rush of relief and endorphins that was genuinely ecstatic, but I couldn't help thinking, "There's gotta be a more pleasant road to enlightenment than this!" And there is. Life is filled with enough suffering, and you may have to deal with some of various kinds in your practice, but there is no need to create suffering intentionally!

You may either sit cross-legged on the floor or in a chair. In the past I was once quite lax in urging proper posture. I indulged my own naturally lazy inclinations and allowed my students to recline however they wished, in big soft, puffy chairs or even to lie down in bed if that seemed best. But this resulted in a lot of people falling asleep while using my meditation tools, and while sleep is great, essential for proper human functioning, it is not the intention of these practices – quite the opposite really. My aim is for you to become more aware of consciousness in its surroundings, and aware of every part of the inner being.

The most important thing is to start by sitting in an upright position that allows you to breathe deeply and fully. You should sit on a meditation pillow or other meditation seat that allows your hips to be slightly elevated. I highly encourage you to sit on the floor rather than a chair. Many modern meditation teachers allow or even encourage students to sit in chairs. There are several reasons why the floor is better. First, sitting on the floor is going to make your meditation practice a different kind of experience from your work life in which you sit in a chair for most of the day in all likelihood. You will immediately be entering a special context and that will help you to get into practice more quickly. Second, and more importantly, the posture of sitting in a chair is not the same as floor sitting. Your hips are more open on the floor and this allows an openness in your awareness that you will not experience in a chair. You will also be able to breathe more deeply and fully. But you can also sit at the edge of a chair as long as it is tall enough that your knees are below the edge.

Many people like to sit on the Zen meditation set up of a *zafu* and *zabuton*. This is a small round pillow on top of a wide flat square pillow. This is an excellent away to practice, but I have spent over ten years developing an even better solution. The challenge with sitting on a small zafu pillow is that no matter what there is going to be a point of contact with the pillow that eventually either causes a painful pressure or a numbness and your legs falling asleep. My current seat is a single surface that has been angled precisely to allow spinal support while spreading the gravitational pressure of sitting across the bottom surface of the legs. I have combined multiple types of padding to create a sitting environment that disappears allowing me to concentrate without any strong bodily distractions whatsoever. I am not sure whether there is a market for this device but if you are interested you should contact me for more information.

Generally speaking though, a proper stable posture will allow you to relax deeply but keep you from becoming too lethargic, sleepy, unfocused. Here is an overview of how to sit properly

Legs

If you do not have any dedicated meditation seat you can sit on a mattress, thick blanket or carpet, and use some firm pillows to support the buttocks. Do not allow the lack of any items to prevent you from beginning. Sit toward the front of the pillow(s), so that the upper hips rotate slightly forward to keep the spine upright.

Although often depicted in books about meditation, sitting in padmasana (the lotus posture) is absolutely not necessary, unless you truly enjoy it. Only a very flexible person can sit in this position and still feel comfortable. Instead, I recommend sitting with knees spread fully resting at your sides with one foot drawn up near your groin and the other foot placed in front of it wherever it feels comfortable. This is generally called sukhasana (enjoyable pose). Some people are not even flexible enough for this posture, and that is one of the reasons for the numerous hip opening postures in the preliminary stretch. Having your hips open is having your essence open and your vital energy open. Work on it.

If you choose to sit in a chair, sit up straight on the edge of the chair. Only the buttocks should be on the chair, with the genitals free (and uncrushed if you are male) at the edge of the chair. Do not lean back on the backrest. Choose a chair that is high enough that the knees can be lower than the hips so that you will not feel an urge to slump backward. A stool can be quite useful in this. Placing a pillow on the chair can reduce strain and pressure on the buttocks.

Back

Keep the spine erect and roll the hips slightly forward if you need to in order to hold the spine up straight comfortably. Gently stretch the spine upward through to the top of the head, as if there is a string attached to the very crown of the head pulling you gently upwards. Then let each vertebra settle on top of the next so that they are stacked neatly in a straight vertical line. Allow the body to fully relax in this position once you are neatly stacked, balancing effortlessly.

Arms

Rest the hands either in the lap or on the thighs. Allow the shoulders to roll back and down into a comfortable and relaxed position, not straining, just relaxing.

Head

Allow the chin to tuck in very slightly (only if this makes the head more comfortable).

Mouth

Relax the jaw. Keep the upper and lower teeth slightly separated.

Tongue

Let the tongue rest against the back of the upper teeth and the palate.

Once you have established this posture you are going to want to stay as still as possible for the remainder of the meditation session. This stillness is an important part of obtaining deeper and deeper awareness of reality and better meditation outcomes. However, if you begin to have some kind of unbearable pain, move as you need to consciously and conscientiously and return to stillness as soon as possible.

Recollection of Intent

Once you have established your stable posture it is important to take a moment to establish the clear purpose why you are sitting for meditation. Think about what level of meditation you are currently working at and set a goal to meet or surpass that level. In other words, if you are at level one, set a clear goal to stay with your meditation object 50% of the time or more.

You may at this time want to think about the enlightened teachers that inspire you and aspire to find your place among them. A form of this is found in Buddhism and called "taking refuge," and you can do this in the formalized Buddhist way if you wish with the three jewels,[5] or you can simply seek to connect with and be supported by the enlightened teachers you admire, living or dead, real or mythological. In my practice I generally connect with a divine white light above me that I know connects me with all possibilities.

After this, take a moment to establish an enlightened intention for your practice. This is sometimes called "Establishing Bodhicitta." You are not practicing meditation just to personally feel good, but to be of service to the world around you. Take a moment to think about the people in your life that you care about, and recognize that when you are an enlightened being you will be able to be much better for them. Imagine how much more you could be good to them and for them if you were a completely enlightened being and make a firm commitment to be fully present in your practice. You can expand this to include all beings everywhere as your enlightened intentions grow over time.

The purpose of this practice is quite practical. It is impossible to obtain enlightenment merely through the desire of the ego to be enlightened. This very ego desire traps us within its own boundaries because even if you achieve some sort of blissful state of trance it will simply gratify and inflate the lower ego, and you will still be trapped within its boundaries.

---

[5] The Three Jewels are The Buddha, The Sangha or enlightened community, and the Dharma or way of Buddhism.

The way out of the problem is quite simple. Instead of attempting to obtain enlightenment for yourself, you direct your energies toward obtaining liberation and complete enlightenment for the sake of all sentient beings in the universe, so that you may be of service and they too may eventually be liberated from suffering and obtain enlightenment for themselves. Your effort is not to force enlightenment or liberation upon others, but rather simply to make oneself available eternally to all who are seeking enlightenment, and to be of whatever assistance you can be. This generosity of purpose will purify your intentions and allow you to eventually become liberated from all delusion. This is not a sacrifice of your True Will, but rather a subjugation of the elements of your lower personality to the purposes of higher consciousness. There is nothing lost, but your consciousness will explode with new potential. It is truly a key that unlocks the gateway to genuine illumination in this lifetime. This illumined consciousness can simply be viewed as a stage of existence in which one is no longer resistant to what "is," in any way. By removing every tension, fear, block, conceptual limitation, description, preconception, stress, desire and aversion one simply exists in the light of pure awareness.

You may also make the firm intention to seek to keep your practice as fresh and new as possible, not merely a habit, keeping in mind that life is short and you never know when your last practice ever will be. You may sit down for meditation practice thousands of times. Make sure each time is a fresh and powerful experience. Always seek a novel experience. Do not let your meditative states become habitual. How can you go deeper today? How can you see more clearly today? How can you be even more focused? Today may lead to an awakening that will change our life forever. Today could also be your very last day on earth, so make this your very best meditation ever. This is your opportunity.

Finally, you can also take a moment to consciously put away any mundane matters that may be on your mind at the time, putting them into a big heavy-lidded imaginary box where you can leave them safely and return to them later after your practice. This simple little mental trick can help immensely if you use it.

Breathing

As mentioned previously, a short period of deep breathing deeply changes your state of consciousness radically and prepares your consciousness for concentration on the meditation object. In the pranayama practices described later n this book, the breathing is the practice, or the gateway to the practice, but I still recommend that you do some deep breathing at the start of even those practices, still followed by the progressive relaxation we will talk about in the next step. This will dramatically increase the oxygen supply in your body. It will allow your heart rate to slow down, calming your body and allow to start relaxing.

You may wish to start by completely emptying the lungs. As you let it out, pull your abdomen inward and upward, fully emptying your lungs.
Then inhale deeply and slowly, drawing the air down deep into your belly, allowing your diaphragm and abdomen to open up completely. Continue to fluidly breathe air in, allowing your ribcage and back to open, and allow the air to fill your lungs all the way up to your collarbone. Your entire lung capacity should be comfortably full. You may even feel a slight pressure in your sinuses when you are totally filled properly, but don't hurt yourself.

Release the breath slowly.

In this, focus slightly more on breathing in than breathing out. Make it your intention to get as much air into your system as possible. Breathe in this manner for between one and five minutes. You will really feel a transformation. If you should start to feel light headed, place your focus down into your belly and intend the energy to move there. This may seem to be a strange statement, but it works surprisingly easily.

Once you have done this, check your posture to make sure you are still upright and supported, and move on to relaxation.

Progressive Relaxation

As with breathing this step is designed to bring you further into the present, further into your body, further into an altered state. Any who are often "stuck in their head," sometimes have a little trouble with this, but it isa very easy and natural process for most people. Basically, all you need to do is go through your body piece by piece, area by area, and release any tension you find there. Start at the top of your head, and work your way down to the toes. While you should make sure you examine every part, the following list represents most of the places where tension can hide.

- Your scalp
- Your forehead and back of head
- Your eyes and your cheeks
- Your jaw
- Your neck
- Your shoulders
- Your arms and hands
- Your upper back and shoulder blades
- Your stomach and lower back
- Your hips
- Your thighs, both front and back
- Your knees
- Your calves
- Your ankles, feet and toes

You do not need to devote a huge amount of time to this process. Simply move your attention to each part and release anything you find there.

The Central Practice

Now you are ready to fully engage the thrupple of attention on your meditation object. A number of different specific practices are described in a later section more detail. Generally, these practices are…

- Focus
- Mantra
- Bhakti
- Breath
- Mindful
- Inquiry

In addition, three transformative pranayama practices are described under the names

- Deep
- Fast
- 1:4:2

You will engage one of these practices for between fifteen minutes and an hour. You will not switch around the practices in the middle or vary between them. Practice only one of these in a sitting.

However, once you become familiar with one, you can work with others too. For instance you could practice Focus on Mondays, Wednesdays and Fridays, and Sundays, while practicing Deep Pranayama on Tuesdays, Thursdays and Saturdays. Or you could work on Fast Pranayama in the morning and Mindful meditation in the evening. These are just examples. You can do as you wish. I do however recommend that you center your practice on one or two of them rather than switching to something different every day. Certainly at first you may wish to do so, in order to see which practices work best with your constitution.

Elevating Emotions

Before concluding your practice you will practice a few more consciousness exercises in order help condition your awareness in a more positive direction, to further refine awareness and to experience pleasant emotions at the end of practice to inspire you to wish to continue.

The basis for this practice is what is called the Brahma-Viharas in some forms of Buddhism, the Four Immeasurables in others and sometimes simply called the practice of Metta. It has also been called Radiating Rosicrucian love in the Western Occult tradition. The basics of the practice are the same in all cases, though some versions are more thorough than others.

There are four states which are identified with the divine realms. These are:

- Loving-kindness (Pali: METTA) good will towards all
- Compassion (Pali: KARUNA) experiencing the suffering of others
- Shared joy (Pali: MUDITA) joy because others are happy
- Equanimity (Pali: UPEKKHA) unshakeable serenity

The *Yoga Sutras* of Patanjali list the exact same qualities in the thirty-third sutra of the first chapter but in Sanskrit rather than Pali.

- MAITRI
- KARUNA
- MUDITA
- UPEKSA

The practice clearly pre-dates Buddhism and plays a part of many different practical spiritual traditions. These elevated feelings are universal feelings of a spiritually advanced person.

At the end of your practice period you will evoke each of these feelings in turn, adding the additional elevated emotions of gratitude and forgiveness at appropriate places within the first two.

LOVING-KINDNESS/GRATITUDE – You will begin by thinking about someone specific that you care about, someone close to you (a parent, a sibling, a child, a lifelong friend or partner, a teacher or mentor) and imagine how much you deeply and purely care about that person. You will allow that pure love to grow stronger and stronger in your heart. Project your love to that person and allow that pure loving energy to flow back to you so that you are basking in loving kindness. Then allow yourself to feel a profound sense of gratitude for this loving kindness in your life and your loved one's life, and gratitude for just being alive.

COMPASSION/FORGIVENESS - Then begin to think about someone specific you care about who is suffering and become vividly aware of how much you would do anything possible to alleviate that suffering. Project that pure compassion to this person and allow it to flow back to you so that you are both basking in compassion. Take moment to forgive this person for any wrong's they may have done you and to allow yourself to be forgiven.

SHARED JOY - Then begin to think about someone specific you care about and imagine how much you take joy in their happiness and success as if it is your own joy. Project this shared joy to that person and allow the joy to flow back to you so that you are basking in it.

EQUANIMITY – Allow a deep sense of centered calm and equilibrium to grow from these feelings, and to know that you will be more and more even tempered and composed as you move forward in your life, with a steady mind, peaceful and serene.

As you develop along your path, you can extend this loving kindness, compassion, joy and equanimity out further and further, so that in a single practice you send it to:

- Someone you are close to
- Your whole community
- Your whole city or region
- Your whole nation
- The whole world
- The whole universe

This way, in every practice session you are sharing these elevated emotions infinitely. It is a wonderful practice because it is positive for you and positive for everyone, everywhere.

The Brahma-Viharas can also form the basis of your whole central practice as a variation on the Bhakti practice you will learn soon, using your special someone as the focal point rather than a divinity. In this case, you will just stay with loving-kindness and allow the other three emotions to develop as a natural result. If you do this Bhakti variation, I still recommend that you conduct the exercise above anyway at the conclusion of your session, as it is a wonderful way to end your practice.

Future Pacing

Studies have shown that mental rehearsal positively affects confidence as well as outcomes. Athletes and performers often practice their routines mentally to give them an edge. You will take advantage of this idea to briefly condition yourself to deal with everyone you meet in the future with these four enlightened emotional reactions.

You simply project your awareness forward into the future, to later in the day, tomorrow and into the future from now on and as you encounter people in your life experience yourself encountering them with the feelings you have just produced. Really get the feeling of experiencing the world in this way. All the people and experiences in your life can be felt with kindness, compassion, joy and equanimity.

You can also take advantage of your currently elevated state to spend a few moments consciously projecting the manifestation of your current plans and visions for the future.

Sharing the Benefits

As you begin all of your practices with generating an enlightened intent you will also end each of your practices by energetically share the benefits with everyone you love or "dedicating the merit" toward the liberation and enlightenment of all beings. By doing this you will seal your practice outside the grasp of your ego-consciousness. The virtue of your endeavor enters the stream of all consciousness, and this prevents your effort from becoming contaminated and swiftly undone by the failings of your lower consciousness.

Just take a moment to freely and energetically share all the wonderful benefits from your practice with everyone you care about or even to be dedicated to the complete liberation and supreme enlightenment of all beings everywhere, and dedicate your energy to improving your relationships with everyone you know.

A Few Meta Tools

There are a number of helping strategies that have been devised over the centuries to make the focusing easier. In an ideal world, we would choose our meditation object, sit down and commune with it perfectly. But the busy mind has other plans, so we can utilize the following with virtually any of the following specific techniques. Where appropriate, they will be mentioned in the tips to follow, but keep in mind that you can add the use of these to any of the meditations to follow.

- Visual Images – such as symbols, shapes, inspiring or divine images
- Counting – usually from one to ten repeatedly
- Prayer Beads – used as a kinesthetic way to count breaths or mantras
- Mantra (Sound Repetition) AUM, HAMSA, SOHAM, IAM, ARAHAN etc.

PART 3 – MEDITATION PRACTICES

There is really only one meditation. There are varying descriptions of how to approach meditation, but ultimately the purpose is singular. There are different styles, vehicles and tools for meditation. There are some misleading instructions and instructors that teach things that do not lead toward meditative states. But meditation itself is simply the art and science of experiencing reality in greater and greater fullness without trying to change, interpret or own it.

The following is not meant to be an exhaustive catalog of all possible meditation styles or tools. Instead it is a collection of the basic categories of these, with a few examples of varieties and then some simple suggestive instructions. I would suggest keeping it simple and utilizing these practices as they are here, but you may also find that you have some other practice that you now understand better thanks to this book and you will use that instead, with the understanding you have gathered here.

Remember, the central instruction of every practice is to continuously and calmly re-center the full thrupple of your attention on the meditation object. We will focus on the various approaches to the thrupple of attention for each practice, and how these slight differences alter the approach but not the destination.

I should also mention again that I have created guided audios for each one of the following specific meditation categories with very open guidance that will allow you to tailor your practice to your own needs. You can find these at jasonaugustusnewcomb.com and elsewhere.

These recordings combine all the above steps including posture, recollection of intent, centering breathwork, progressive relaxation, the central practice, open awareness, elevated emotions, future pacing, and sharing the benefits.

Each of the following practices emphasizes the thrupple of attention in slightly different ways, with greater focus on one or more of the senses, and with different levels of focus in general. Experiment with all of them to see which practice fits your personal consciousness best.

You will want to use your whole attention for this work, conscious and subconscious, foveal and peripheral. You are going to want to hold several things in attention at once. This should not be done forcefully, but rather just diligently. Your attention will flag and stray pretty regularly. Just return it to the task at hand when you notice that you have drifted. Make sure that you take a moment to feel good for noticing that you have wandered, rather than feeling bad for mind wandering. It is possible to get distracted for long periods. Your goal is to shorten these and eventually to be able to focus with unbroken attention. The only way to train your mind is to reward the noticing. Rewarding the noticing makes your awareness recognize that the goal is concentration. Punishing the wandering is only going to make your mind wander more because until you notice it the wandering goes unpunished and so your awareness will keep wandering and never let you notice to avoid punishment.

You may also begin to "zone out." Don't let this happen. Maintain a lucid focus on the energy you are working with, in the ways explained below. The good news is that when focusing on several things at once it is actually easier to maintain awareness because you are not leaving as much room for distracting elements and lethargy to gain a foothold in your awareness. Make sure that you keep your practice fresh by really focusing as vividly as possible on all the colors, feelings, sounds, energies and process every time, and making it your intention to do it more and more deeply and effectively each time.

Focus

Focus meditation guides you to use any object as your focal point, a candle flame, a crystal, a statue, a shape, and focus your complete attention upon it visually and kinesthetically while describing with a single meaningful word such as "flame" or "heat." Eventually the process yields to fixation and transcendence into the eternal now.

The first three practices we will discuss are really inter-related and may end up resembling each other in some ways. The key difference with each of them is the sensory channel that forms the main focus of practical awareness, with the other two acting as supportive partners in the thrupple of attention.

With the Focus practice, the leading sense is visual. That classic image of a holy person staring intently at a candle flame is an example of one version of the Focus meditation practice. In this practice you choose an object to look at or to visualize with your inner eye, and maintain a concentrated awareness on that visual object.

There are many different variations on this practice. Theravada Buddhists will stare at simple mandalas they call *kasina*. Yogis will stare at a flame, at the setting sun, mandalas or *yantras* which are geometric shapes sacred to various deities. As far as more internalized practices go, Yogis will visualize elemental shapes called *tattwas*, or various deities associated with elements, chakras, or both. Tibetan Buddhists will visualize complex deities. The possibilities are really endless, and for practical purposes you simply need to choose something that appeals to you.

You can do whatever you want, but to keep things easy I will give the example of, and recommend utilizing, one of the five ancient elements, earth, water, fire, air and ether or space. You can use a symbolic representation, a physical sample, a chakra or point in your body, or a combination, as long as it is simple and singular. For instance, you can visualize a red triangle in your belly as a fire Focus, or you could visualize a flame in your belly, or you could visualize either out in front of you. You could also have a physical representation of either and look at it with eyes open.

Earth – yellow square – lump of clay or stone – perineum
Water – silver crescent – cup of water – sexual orgrans
Fire – red triangle – candle flame – navel area
Air – grey hexagram – incense smoke - chest
Ether – black egg – sky – throat

Any one of these could be your chosen object. Make sure you choose one as the main practice focus and stick with it until you experience a complete absorption state on that object. However, the full thrupple of attention must be engaged as follows.

Thrupple of Attention:

Visual: an object that you look at physically or mentally
Auditory: the inner sound of a word describing the object, its qualities or a mantra
Kinesthetic: physical sensation of the point of contact with the breath

For the auditory component of the elements you could simply repeat the name of the element in English or your preferred language, or you could repeat the name in Sanskrit or Pali, or a *bija mantra* of the element, as follows in this order below.

Earth – PRITHIVI – PATAVI – LAM (LANG)
Water – APAS – APO – VAM (VANG)
Fire – TEJAS – TEJO – RAM (RANG)
Air – VAYU – VAYU – YAM (YANG)
Ether – AKASHA – AKASA – HAM (HANG)

As far as the kinesthetic sensations of the elements go, the following are some of the simplest and most practical sensations to focus upon.

Earth – mass, heaviness, solidity
Water – volume, fluidity, viscosity
Fire – temperature, heat, light
Air - motion, flow, insubstantiality
Ether – infinite expanse

Obviously, you are not restricted to the elements at all. You can utilize whatever object you wish, as long as you can associate a sound and emotion or kinesthetic feeling to it. You can utilize more complex chakra images, deity images or any other object as long as you can engage the full thrupple.

An advanced variation on this practice is to simply focus your visual attention with open awareness at one of the areas of your body, most usually the third eye or the tip of the nose. The entire practice becomes one of open experience rather than controlled concentration. I recommend developing the concentration first.

The Practice:

After establishing your posture and the other preparatory processes through progressive relaxation you will begin to focus your attention on the visual object you have chosen. At first simply be aware of the object as it rests in relation to you, either physically or mentally. Then begin to feel the object kinesthetically and finally begin to silently repeat your descriptive word or mantra. As your attention flags or wanders congratulate yourself for noticing and return to the visual image and then the rest of the thrupple.

Tips:

- This practice centers initially on the visual, but you want to powerfully engage all three senses.

- A physical object or image is often easier to work with than a purely mental construct. You can close your eyes and continue to visualize, or else simply continue to stare at the object throughout.

- Prepare yourself for many visual distortions whether you are working with closed or open eyes. Simply remain focused and return to the object when you can.

- You may wish to add counting 1-10 between mantras or descriptive words if you find your attention flagging too quickly. Use this only as "training wheels" and discard the counting as soon as you are stabilized.

Mantra

As Focus meditation begins with the visual, Mantra begins with the auditory. Mantra meditation focuses on the silent repetition of a sacred sound over and over again. This process allows you to focus deeply on the experience and tune in to the frequency of the infinite.

Mantra meditation was one of the earliest popular meditation imports from India, in the form of Maharishi Mahesh Yogi's Transcendental Meditation movement in the sixties which had a huge impact on the conscious living movement. However, mantra meditation is a worldwide phenomenon that really does not have anything to do with eastern mysticism at all. Many Christian mystics over the centuries have simply repeated the word "God," as a mantra. This simple practice can be traced to the twelfth century or earlier within Christianity. The repetition of sacred words is a universal technique for centering awareness in the present moment. You will discover a deep sacred bliss with the use of mantra meditation.

People use many different mantras in practice. AUM, IAM, HAMSA, SOHAM as well as the bija mantras of the chakras are some of the most common. You may use any of these or one given to you by a guru, or even your TM mantra with this technique. You can also use the name of your God if you have one and that seems appropriate to you. The only important caveat is that you use just one for your whole practice, and that you center your practice around the same mantra in general.

Thrupple of Attention:

Auditory: the inner mental sound of the mantra
Kinesthetic: the subtle vibration of the mantra, feeling of the mantra, power of the mantra
Visual: open awareness, a sacred image, light, or the third eye, also perineum

Visually concentrating the mantra into a specific bodily location and feeling its vibration there is a powerful method of engaging the full thrupple of attention. The third eye, or space between the eyes is a classic spot for this, as well as the perineum which is often considered the resting place of Kundalini. The heart is also an excellent place to focus your mantra.

An advanced variation on this practice that you may wish to engage at some time in the future is to not make an inner sound but instead to listen inside yourself for the subtle inner sounds or Nadas. This is most often done at the heart center, though the sounds may emanate from elsewhere.

The Practice:

After establishing your posture and the other preparatory processes through progressive relaxation simply focus your attention on the mantra of your choice. If you do not have a mantra that you have been given or that you feel drawn to, I recommend using "AUM," the classic mantra of mantras. Feel the subtle vibration of the mentally formed mantra. Let the mantra repeat fast or slow in your awareness. While doing so you can either have your visual attention open on experiencing your whole body, or focused on some particular spot. Do not try time or control your mantra with your breathing. If it happens that is fine. Just experience it openly. As your attention flags or wanders congratulate yourself for noticing and return to the mantra and then the rest of the thrupple.

Tips:

- You may use any seed mantra you wish for this. You can just use OM or one provided by a teacher as well.

- Using a short "seed" mantra is probably best.

- You may wish to add counting 1-10 between mantras if you find your attention flagging too quickly. Use this only as "training wheels" and discard the counting as soon as you are stabilized.

- Engage the visual and kinesthetic as well.

Bhakti

To round out the senses, Bhakti meditation centers its focus on the feelings and sensations, particularly the feeling of loving devotion to the divine. Bhakti meditation is a form of meditation that is based on devotion with deep love and a direct divine experience. It is a method meditation that greatly rewards your dedication. It is often considered the fastest and best meditation method for those who are religious. The commentary in the *Yoga Sutras* of Pantanjali describes one way of approaching this type of meditation in which you repeat AUM while focusing upon *Isvara*. The Christian mystical book *The Cloud of Unknowing* describes a similar approach where you say "God" over and over while giving yourself completely to him. There are several Buddhist meditations that offer variations involving deities of various types. These may seem different in religious sentiment, but they all center around a love for the divine.

This type of meditation is often considered the fastest method of experiencing deep meditation. Sometimes this is explained as a product of the blessing of your God or Goddess. Other times it is simply explained that the deep emotion creates a powerful vessel of transformation.

Thrupple of Attention:

Kinesthetic: A loving feeling of devotion and desire to deeply connect with the divine
Visual: A divine image
Auditory: The name of the divine being repeated over and over, or a related mantra

The essence of the practice is simply centering yourself on the feeling of divine love. While it is important to have a visual component for the thrupple of attention, if you do not have a specific image in mind I recommend focusing on a globe of light as this is a universal divine symbol. You could also just have an open visual awareness.

If you are not a religious person, but would like to get the advantage of this meditation's inherent power, you may wish to focus on the transcendent love of nature or the natural world. Form a beautiful image of an inspiring landscape, and use the feelings this inspires as the feeling for the meditation. Images such as a starry night sky, a majestic mountain or valley, the ocean, or a forest clearing might evoke that sense of love that is the key to this practice.

It is also possible to focus on a human person, a friend, teacher, mentor or guru, and conduct this practice based upon the love and goodwill you have toward them. This meditation on loving kindness toward someone you care about is a way to conduct the Brahma-Viharas as your whole practice. Let yourself focus on the loving kindness aspect and let the others develop as spontaneous extensions as you experience absorption in these feelings. Obviously you will make the image of your loved one the focal component, and for the auditory you can either mentally say their name repeatedly, or something like, "May you always enjoy love and happiness (name of your loved one)."

The Practice:

After establishing your posture and the other preparatory processes through progressive relaxation focus your attention on the specific divinity you are focusing upon, letting that feeling of loving devotion fill you. Visualize the divine image as needed to inspire that feeling, but center the majority of your focus on the divine feeling. As you repeat a word or name you do not necessarily need to treat it as a mantra, although you can, as long as the mantra inspires the feeling.
As your attention flags or wanders congratulate yourself for noticing and return to the divine and your love for it and the rest of the thrupple.

Tips:

- This type of practice utilizes components of some of the other methods and may seem to be quite similar. The distinct difference is in that devotional loving energy that is unique to love of a divine personage.

- You could easily just visualize light as the image if your divinity does not have a form, or if you would prefer a more formless divine experience, either a sphere of light or just a general brightness

- Make the center of the practice the feeling of divine love.

- Let whatever visual image you are using be simply be an inspiration toward love.

- You can use a physical image or statue to focus upon visually if you wish.

- Rather than repeating the divine name over and over, you may just wish to say it occasionally to help keeping focused on that divine sense of love.

- You may wish to add counting 1-10 between mantras if you find your attention flagging too quickly. Use this only as "training wheels" and discard the counting as soon as you are stabilized.

- As mentioned above, this type of meditation can also be practiced as a Metta or Brahma-Vihara meditation that fills the whole session. Simply get a feeling of loving kindness for a special person, visualize them, and say either "loving kindness" or the person's name over and over to engage the full thrupple.

Breath

Breath meditation focuses your attention on the process of respiration, allowing an extremely portable and entirely secular technique that grows quickly into deep states of bliss. Like Bhakti, it focuses around feelings, but now specifically the kinesthetic feelings of respiration.

Mindfulness of breathing is one of the most commonly taught meditation strategies today. There are a number of slight variations but in practice they are basically the same process. Zen Buddhism and Theravada Buddhism use breath awareness as a primary technique. But you don't need to be a Buddhist to practice this way. Even completely secular meditation programs like Mindfulness Based Stress Relief (MBSR) use breath awareness. However, breath awareness is in fact also the meditation method that is most associated the enlightenment of the historical Buddha. However, that practice was really more like the next one we will discuss. But simply attending to the breath can focus your mind into absorption surprisingly quickly.

It is an extremely simple and yet powerful method of calmly centering awareness in the present moment in order to silence the wandering mind and enter into bliss. Even though this technique is fairly simple, it is extremely transformative.

Thrupple of Attention:

Kinesthetic: physical sensation of the point of contact with the breath
Visual: inner impression of the point of contact with breath
Auditory: open awareness, and any audible sounds of the breath, also counting or other internal verbalization

The Practice:

After establishing your posture and the other preparatory processes through progressive relaxation focus your attention on the breath as it goes in and out. Do not try to alter or control your breathing. Just experience it however it is moving. Focus on the sensations where the air meets your upper lip and nostrils. As your attention flags or wanders congratulate yourself for noticing and return your awareness to the thrupple of attention at the point of contact with the breath.

Tips:

- In order to more fully engage the thrupple, you may wish initially to count your breaths in your mind as you go, at least at first. This way you are engaging the auditory, visual and kinesthetic senses together. Generally it is suggested that you count to ten and then return to one again. This serves two purposes. It keeps the count from growing confusing, but also checks the tendency to go on mental auto pilot. If you count eleven you will know you have not been attending well.

- You can also utilize a mantra such as OM with each breath. The mantra HAMSA or SOHAM is naturally tuned to the breath, with the "S" syllable formed by the in breath and the "H" syllable on the out breath.

- The visual component can be engaged by just gently attending to the area where you are feeling sensations. You don't need to visualize anything specific, just allow your visual awareness to center on the spots where the breath gently tickles your nose and face.

- In order to keep your interest, you may wish to see how deeply and in how detailed you can observe the breathing sensations.

- You may also wish to observe the movements in your belly rather than the nose. However, you should not try to do both because this will be agitating and not conducive to your deepening meditation.

- Make sure you are engaging the full thrupple of your attention on the practice, even if it is just focused open awareness with the visual and auditory components.

Mindful

With the Mindful practice, we equally engage all three parts of the thrupple, but with an entirely open approach. Mindfulness is the hottest term in meditation today. While breath awareness is the most commonly prescribed form of mindfulness, the mindful practice actually encompasses a full awareness of the whole field of perception, particularly focusing on the four foundations of mindfulness, BODY, FEELINGS, THOUGHTS, and the PROCESS OF EXPERIENCE or DHARMA in Buddhist terminology. Of great importance in the practice is noticing that all four are just objects of awareness or experiences that come and go. If any one of them disappeared forever it would not take away any of your personal sense. None of these four are your "self."

This can be conducted in a number of different ways, but each approach really centers around a present awareness of the experience you are having in the moment. This places the practitioner into a simply open experience of what is happening. Rather than pushing anything away, you simply allow yourself to watch, listen and feel whatever is happening without holding onto any of it. Eventually, complete tranquility and lucid awareness melt into bliss and equanimity.

This experience is the open awareness that I have been describing here and there throughout these practices. So, in essence your purpose is to simply be aware of the experience of being, as completely as possible.

Thrupple of Attention:

Visual: open awareness
Auditory: open awareness
Kinesthetic: open awareness

Mindful meditation focuses your attention in more of an open manner upon the totality of your experience. Various specific Buddhist methods such as the body scan, noting, breath awareness, *vipassana, samatha, satipatthana, zazen, samadhi, jhana, panna,* and *anapanasati* as well as other practices utilize this stategy but in this practice you will explore this simply and powerfully to uncover the bliss that lies behind phenomenal experience.

This is the most open of the meditations and this can make it very relaxing and powerful, but it can also be easier to get distracted. Keep your attention centered on the body, simply aware of other stuff that comes up as it happens but keeping focus primarily on the body. You can do this centering on your body by feeling everything all at once holistically, or you can slowly move through your body piece by piece, up and down as in the first part of the recording.

The Practice:

After establishing your posture and the other preparatory processes through progressive relaxation continue to focus your attention on (BODY) your body and the breath going in and out. Focus on the physicality of the body, the flesh and bones, moving from head to feet. Recognize very consciously that no particular part of the body is yourself... none of its components all the way down to its atoms are actually you... (FEELING) And move awareness to the feelings and notice that pleasant and unpleasant feelings arise and disappear all throughout the body, and none are you. There is not one permanent feeling, and no feeling is you. (THOUGHTS) And move awareness to the thought processes and recognize that thoughts are fleeting experiences that come and go, and are either related to desires or to fears, or else are just random noise, and recognize very consciously that no particular thought is yourself. (PROCESS/DHARMA) And then continue to experience an open awareness of your body, feelings, thoughts and the process of awareness itself, noticing your body from head to toes as one thing, an object in your awareness, the feelings that flow, any thoughts that pass by and the whole experience of awareness. And keep your attention on the open experience of everything in your awareness. As your attention flags or wanders congratulate yourself for noticing and return your awareness to an open awareness of thrupple of attention.

Tips:

- The thrupple of attention is completely open ended in this form, so it may be a bit of challenge for meditators with extremely restless minds. However, by allowing yourself to relax more and more deeply you will find that restlessness disappears.

- Likewise, for overly lethargic meditators this meditation can be one that is easy to sleep through. Ay of the following can be used to avoid this.

- You can repeatedly move your attention over your body piece by piece as an approach.

- You can make a quick mental note of anything that comes up in awareness.

- You can move through the foundations of body, feelings, thoughts and process over and over again.

- Whatever choice you make, stick with it for the whole meditation period as much as possible.

- This meditation engages kinesthetics well, but you must be a bit creative when it comes to auditory and visual focus. You can "see" your body from the inside, but make sure this is a real visual engagement and not a day dream that takes you out of your actual present experience. For sound, you can list what you are experiencing, you can count breaths (1-10), or you could even use a mantra. This latter is not necessary, but if you find your thoughts constantly wandering can be a last resort. Use this only as "training wheels" and discard the counting as soon as you are stabilized.

Inquiry

Inquiry meditation inverts the whole process in on itself. It is both the easiest and most challenging of the techniques. It is sometimes called the direct method, since it focuses directly on the experiencer, rather than any object in experience. Inquiry meditation asks the question, "who is the experiencer?" and directs you to experience you in this present moment, outside of anything you are experiencing. Who are you?

It is in many ways the mirror of the Mindful technique, and its natural conclusion, but approached directly. In this technique you focus on the simple fact that everything experienced is not you. It is just an experience. There is an experiencer who is having the experience and this experiencer is separate from any object it is experiencing. Even the sensations of the body are not you. They are sensations. The experiencer can locate sensations, but is not those sensations. Thoughts are not you. They are experiences. In this technique you simply move your attention to the experiencer and hold it here. Experience what happens as you hold awareness on itself.

You are outside of space and time. You are not an experience of various objects. You are unbounded, eternal, clear and radiant. The fastest and easiest way to experience this directly is simply to look inward and discover who the experiencer is. What you see, hear, feel, taste and touch is not it. These are just experiences, not the experiencer. So, while you may experience these, dive deeper within, turning instead toward that which is experiencing. What you think and the stream of thoughts is not it, these too are just experiences. Dive deeper. What you consider yourself, your desires, labels, fears, doubts and every other occurrence in your awareness on any level is not it. Visions of angels or the throne of God are not it. No experience is the experience. You just are. Get this directly and you are enlightened. It's that simple.

Thrupple of Attention:

Visual: inverted back upon the seer
Auditory: inverted back upon the hearer
Kinesthetic: inverted back upon the feeler

The Practice:

After establishing your posture and the other preparatory processes through progressive relaxation focus your attention on the experiences in awareness briefly, then turn the experiencer in on itself. Who is experiencing this awareness? No object, label, or sensation is it. These are experiences. Focus on the experiencer. As your attention flags or wanders congratulate yourself for noticing and return your awareness to an open awareness of thrupple of attention.

Tips:

- As experiences come into awareness in any part of the thrupple, immediately turn attention around inward from the experience, seeking who is experiencing this.

- Initially you may find you are focusing on subtle experiences rather than awareness. Do not get distracted and continue diving inward.

- You may ask the question, "Who am I?" or "What is the Experiencer?" but only do so sincerely. Don't make it a sing-song or mantra.

Pranayama Practices

Before concluding I want to share a few breathing techniques that while perhaps technically not meditation practices, share both the same purpose and potentially the same result as the meditations, but coming from an energetic perspective. As mentioned previously, deep breathing has at least two naturally amazing effects on consciousness. One, it encourages the relaxation response physiologically, and two, it naturally bridges and connects the conscious and unconscious parts of our awareness. Further, breathing deeply improves cellular metabolism, improves circulation and general health. Breathing in specific ways also has the capacity to make extremely profound shifts in awareness, and feelings of energies swirling powerfully in the body. These profound energy experiences are most frequently called *Prana Shakti* or *Kundalini Shakti*. As mentioned before we are not going to focus on the metaphysical concepts. Instead we are going to focus on powerful techniques that deliver undeniable results that do not depend on any particular belief system. The three practices we are going to explore I call:

Deep Pranayama
Fast Pranayama
1:4:2 Pranayama

Pranayama forms a very central role in the Hatha Yoga tradition, but does not get nearly as much attention from modern exponents as the postural positions that actually have a much smaller role in the early tradition. Breath is also greatly important to Tibetan Buddhism, which has a strong yogic component. The purpose of pranayama is generally twofold. One, it is to purify the subtle energetic nerve system called "the nadis." Secondly, it is to move the breath energies, often through inner heat, in some form of process to awaken Kundalini.

As you explore the techniques in the coming pages you are going to notice a few things without doubt. One, you are going to feel greater personal focus, greater personal energy, more tranquility, you are going to find your sinuses clearer, and your breathing deeper. This is cleansing "the nadis." Two, you are going to experience profound energy flows, and discover that you can direct these flows with your attention and some subtle physical prompting. If you devote serious time to these practices, you will discover that it is possible to collapse the perception of the physical universe just with breathing. You don't have to do anything but breathe and focus your attention.

There are a large number of pranayama practices, some books are filled with dozens of them, and I am going to share only three. Why? Because I believe these three form the core of nearly everything essential related to the transformative aspects of pranayama. Also, I offer a number of variations on how you focus the breath energy so there are really quite a lot more possible practices that you can build by putting different parts together.

Before getting started I want to mention that all of the postural instructions from the earlier section still apply. For that matter, I highly suggest that you conduct these breathing exercises as the central practice within the eight part system described in this book. The only thing that I would add to the previous instructions is that when you are breathing intensely it is highly important that you wear very loose fitting or highly elastic clothing that makes deep breathing comfortable and does not impede blood flow at all.

Let's start laying out the parts.

To begin with, in all three forms of pranayama we will explore I want you to breathe as absolutely deeply and fully as you can with every breath. I want you to breathe into your diaphragm, your back, your chest, everything that you've got. Breathe as deeply as possible, filling yourself up throughout. Do not hurt yourself, but try to fill the bottom of your belly all the way to your top of your nasal passages with every breath. Fill your lungs right to the edge of discomfort if possible, but not to where you are actually uncomfortable. Maximize your oxygen draw. When you are doing this right you will know it because after a minute or two you will start experience tingling at the extremities, flows of inner energy, maybe even some colorful inner lights, and possibly some light headedness. This latter can be avoided if you lightly focus on keeping the energy in your torso.

Whenever you are breathing I want you to focus on breathing in, on drawing breath energy in, more than letting it out. If you fill up early, hold it in at absolutely full rather than letting it out early. In all ways behave as if you are cherishing and hoarding that breath.

You want to be breathing through your nostrils in these practices as much as possible, although if you have a lot of congestion it is okay to use your mouth once in a while. I say this only because, again, I want to emphasize that you are wanting to be taking in the maximum possible oxygen. You may find that congestion clears after a round or two of pranayama. Using your mouth of course makes alternate nostril work impossible, and changes the energy pathways a bit in general.

Let the breathing be as vigorous as necessary to fill to capacity every time, but otherwise relax your body as fully as possible throughout. If you notice tension building up, for instance in your shoulders or arms, try your best to release it. Hold your posture as stably as possible but allow whatever movement is necessary to maximize breath intake.

The kinesthetic and subjective sensation we are going to call breath energy is a real and palpable experience that you can cultivate right now. This breath energy can be flowed in your body in a number of different ways, with different effects. The process of moving the energy has two components.

First and foremost, it is a matter of attention and intention. Wherever your mind focuses your inner sense of awareness the sensations of breath energy are going to grow. Let's do a simple experiment. Put down tyis book for a moment and take ten very profoundly deep breaths just as described above. Count them out on your fingers. When you are done hold your breath and you will notice that there are a number of new flowing and tingling sensations in your body. Observe the sensations for a moment, then begin to concentrate on your left hand, willing this tingly energy to flow there. Congratulations, you just learned to move your energy.

The second component involves some physical contractions and postures that will facilitate containing and moving this energy more precisely where you want it to go, which is into the spinal column through the perineum. These physical movements are of key importance to Hatha Yoga, but very few seem to understand how they work. I will outline them below.

Mula Bandha

This is the root lock. It is pulling up on the perineal region. Some authorities say it should just be the perineum, others include the anal and pubic muscles. You can try either or both. The important thing is to have the felt sense that you are holding and supporting the energy space of your torso so that you can contain and lift the "downward flowing energy." Imagine that your innards might fall out of the bottom of you unless you hold them in a bit. This does not need to be a strong squeeze. Just a gentle upward contraction will suffice.

Uddiyana Bandha

This is the belly lock. It is pulling up and in on your belly muscles. If you look at yogis doing it on video they are often practically touching their spines with their navels. You do not need to do this for this technique. All you need is a gentle containing action of your abdominal muscles. Imagine that your innards might fall out of your belly unless you hold them in a bit.

Jalandhara Bandha

This is the throat lock. Again, we are going to use it only very gently. Just close your throat lightly, and drop your head loosely to your chest. Again, you are just gently containing, trying to make sure the air doesn't float up out of you. The important things is to have the felt sense that you are holding and pushing downward the energy space of your chest and shoulders so that you can contain and push the "upward flowing energy" (prana) into your core.

There are two additional gestures or seals called mudras that I tend to use from traditional Hatha, though I am not absolutely certain that they are completely essential to the process.

Kecari Mudra

This mudra is sticking your tongue toward the back and roof of your mouth. Just do it to the point where you are comfortable. If you can touch the soft palate or nasal passages that is great, but as long as your tongue is making a connection with the roof of your mouth you will be on track.

Gyana Mudra

This mudra is the index fingers and thumbs connecting, with hands resting on thighs. This is pretty much the iconic yogi posture. You can also use the New Hermetics meditation anchor finger positions.

Kumbhaka

Each of the pranayama practices to follow involves periods of breath retention that are traditionally called "kumbhaka." During these periods of breath retention you will engage the three bandhas and two key mudras, doing so gently, allowing your whole body to be otherwise totally and completely relaxed. The kumbhaka practice is exactly the same in all three forms. This may seem a bit complicated but it is actually quite simple and natural.

When you are about to do the kumbhaka portion of the practice you exhale completely, then inhale deeply through both nostrils visualizing the breath energy flowing down the sides of your body down into your belly. As it is flowing in and down you lightly engage mulabandha, pulling energy up to meet the breath in the belly. Then push all this energy down and back toward the spine past the lightly tensed perineum by engaging uddiyana bandha. Then, as you are completely filled with breath engage jalandhara bandha to as you compress everything into your spinal column and concentrate on what is going on in and around your spine and the rest of your torso.

Focus the full thrupple of attention on your spinal column, particularly at the base for now.[6] If you have done this right it will start to become a pretty profoundly ecstatic experience in two to three rounds of practice.

With this essential component explained, let's take a look at each of the practices in turn.

---

[6] Later you can concentrate on the heart center or brow center if you wish, but this not a good idea until you have some experience with directing the spinal energy.

Deep Pranayama

Deep Pranayama focuses on deep and powerful in and out breathing that rapidly increases the energy flowing in your body and assists in arousing transformative energy experiences.

The practice is fairly simple and direct. You will breathe in and out for approximately five seconds each, as deeply as possible, just as described earlier. After around thirty[7] such breaths in a row, you will practice a kumbhaka as described above. You will hold your breath for as long as possible, up to a minute and a half or even more if you wish. Your ability to hold your breath will be significantly extended by the breaths you have been breathing so deeply.

During the period of retention engage the three bandhas and kecari mudra as we went over, doing it gently so that only enough pressure is applied to establish a sense of containment, otherwise allowing your whole body to be totally and completely relaxed.

After retention you can take a few regular breaths, or you can do a second retention. Again, breathe as absolutely deeply as possible at all times.

This process takes approximately five minutes and can be repeated three or more times as much as time allows.

You will discover a lot of profound shifts happening as you explore this. Throughout, you will engage the thrupple of attention in this way.

Thrupple of Attention:

Visual: visualizing the energies flowing in one of the directions as described below
Auditory: open awareness, mantra or counting
Kinesthetic: feeling the movement of the visualized energies

---

[7] 27 is traditional for numerological reasons.

Fast Pranayama

Fast Pranayama focuses on fast and powerful deep breathing at a rapid pace which swiftly clears blockages in your energy system to allow energy to flow more freely. This is especially useful in breaking up old patterns that may be holding you from growing into your full awesomeness.

There are several slightly variant traditional pranayama practices that utilize fast breathing as a tool. There is Bhastrika or the bellows breath, There is Kapalapati or skull shining breath, and Agni Pran, the breath of fire. Some teachers consider all of these the same practice. Some teachers lay out distinctions. Other teachers contradict those distinctions. The important issue is that fast and powerful breathing increases the inner heat in your body, increases the amount of free breath energy that is coursing through your system, and allows you to blast through blockages in your system pretty quickly.

The specific variation we will be using is slightly different from most variations on this practice that I have encountered elsewhere because as with the previous practice we will be focusing on accumulating oxygen even though we are breathing rapidly. The in and out breaths are going to be slightly slower than you usually experience in these fast, fiery, breath techniques. Your in breath should take a little over one second, with your out breath exhaled a bit faster. Because of this you really must use your belly as a bellows in order to powerfully draw in your full capacity of breath, and then to quickly push it back out vigorously. This can all be a bit of a work out for your core abdominal muscles and you may even find yourself losing a pound or two if you regularly use this breath. Allow the process to be vigorous so that you really are getting a massive amount of breath in each time.

After around one hundred[8] such breaths in a row, you will practice a kumbhaka as described above. You will hold your breath for as long as possible, up to a minute and a half or even more if you wish. Your ability to hold your breath will be significantly extended by the breaths you have been breathing so deeply.

---

[8] 108 is traditional for numerological reasons.

During the period of retention engage the three bandhas and kecari mudra as we went over, doing it gently so that only enough pressure is applied to establish a sense of containment, otherwise allowing your whole body to be totally and completely relaxed.

After retention you can take a few regular breaths, or you can do a second retention. Again, breathe as absolutely deeply as possible at all times.

This process takes approximately five minutes and can be repeated three or more times as much as time allows.

Throughout, you will engage the thrupple of attention just as before.

Thrupple of Attention:

Visual: visualizing the energies flowing in one of the directions as described below
Auditory: open awareness, mantra or counting
Kinesthetic: feeling the movement of the visualized energies

1:4:2 Pranayama

1:4:2 Pranayama is an advanced breathing technology that focuses on deep breathing and extended periods of breath retention (kumbhaka) while concentrating the breath energy into the spine. This advanced technology can be explored using alternate nostril breathing (anuloma), breathing through one nostril (surya or chandra), or through both nostrils. Because this practice contains many more periods of Kumbhaka than the other two, you may find it very powerful or very difficult.

This practice is slightly different than the other two. I have saved this practice for last because it is the most complex, and possibly most powerful, though only if you are doing it correctly.

This is one of the most commonly described forms of pranayama in the early literature of Hatha Yoga. It is often conducted along with alternate nostril breathing but not always. The basic structure of the breath is that your inhale or puraka occupies one unit of time, your kumbhaka occupies four of those units, and your exhale or rechaka occupies two units of time.

This can be expanded indefinitely…

Puraka 4 seconds, kumbhaka 16 seconds, rechaka 8 seconds
Puraka 8 seconds, kumbhaka 32 seconds, rechaka 16 seconds
Puraka 16 seconds, kumbhaka 64 seconds, rechaka 32 seconds
And so on.

My recordings utilize a ratio of 6 seconds on inhale (puraka), 24 seconds of retaining (kumbhaka) and 12 seconds of exhale (rechaka). This is probably a good target for most people. You may even find it a bit challenging for a while.

To make it easier I recommend "priming the system" with about ten deep breaths, as in the Deep pranayama technique followed by a few rounds of 1:4:2 pranayama and then some more deep breathing, and some more rounds of 1:4:2 pranayama then more deep breathing and so on so that while you are exploring the edges with purifying kumbhaka you are continuing to care for your safety and not causing any unnecessary suffering. This is how the practice is organized on my recordings.

You may also wish to silently intone "AUM" during the retentions. This instruction can be found I many of the older traditional texts. You may also wish to vibrate this "AUM" in your perineum area.

Throughout, you will engage the thrupple of attention like this.

Thrupple of Attention:

Visual: visualizing the energies flowing in one of the directions as described below
Auditory: open awareness, mantra or counting
Kinesthetic: feeling the movement of the visualized energies

Breathing Visualization Patterns

At first, it is probably a good idea to simply conduct the breathing exercises and get used to the structure of them. Concentrate on the energy movement part only at the kumbhaka section. However, once you have familiarized yourself with the routine, the following visualizations will add significantly to the experiences of all three types of breathing. They can all be used with all three, although Fast pranayama may pose some difficulties with the more intricate visualizations and may be better with the last two, full body visualizations.

Each of these breath variations involves utilizing the thrupple of attention to focus the breath energy as it moves through us in various ways. You will visualize and feel the breath moving along the specified paths as vividly as possible. at the same time you will either count breaths, use a mantra, or both. AUM is often suggested, or HAMSA as described earlier.

For each of these experiences you can visualize the breath energy as some specific color that resonates with you, or else just as a beautiful bluish white radiance.

Alternate Nostril Breathing

In this breath variation you draw the breath energy on one side sending it all the way down to your perineum, then send it up the other side. On the next breath you switch. So you could start by breathing in through your right nostril, then breathing out through your left nostril. Then you breathe in through your left and out through your right. As you breathe in, visualize the breath energy flowing from your nostril down the side of your throat, then through an energy tunnel down the side of your spine leading to the base. The breath is gathered at the perineum each time, either way. To gather it, gently contract the mulabandha. You can physically seal off the unused nostril with a finger if you wish, but it is just as effective just to focus mentally on each nostril rather than blocking anything completely. This methd greatly balances the right and left hemispheres and helps to powerfully train the energy flow into your perineal region which is helpful in the kumbhakas.

You may experiment with using only one nostril for the whole period. When using the right nostril this is Surya breath. With the left nostril this is Chandra breath.

You may also practice this with both nostrils without alternating the nostrils, just sending breath energy down both side columns beside your spine simultaneously. In this case you may wish to experiment with sending the energy up the central column on the exhale. This is a good rehearsal for the kumbhaka segment of these practices in general.

Microcosmic Orbit

In this variation, visualize that the breath flows down to the pit of the belly, and circulates around the genitals, up the back and into the head. Then as you exhale send it down the front of your body to your belly where it is stored. The easiest way to do this is to breathe in pulling the breath energy from the belly down through the groin using mulabhanda and uddiyana bandha to pull it up the spine to the crown, and as you breathe out pushing the energy down through your throat and chest just mov your head as needed to direct the energy back to your belly where it is stored.

This type of movement gives you a sense of grounded power in the gut. It is good for building up your personal sense of inner strength, healing and calm. It balances the energetic sensations and expands your personal force.

Perineum to Crown

With this you pull up lightly on your perineum with the mulabandha as you inhale, as if you were breathing up through your perineum into your spine sort of like sucking a straw. You may involve the other bandhas if they feel useful to the process. You send this visualized and felt energy up the center of your spine to your crown. As you exhale you relax the perineum and send the energy down the spine back to your base.

There is a slight variation of this in which you send the energy from the perineum to third eye instead, and back down as before. It is exactly the same as the previous except that you deviate to the third eye rather than up to the crown.

Another variation can be conducted with either of the last two but circling back down behind the spine. This is the same basic move as the last two except that instead of sending the energy back down the center of the spine as it came up, instead you send it over the top of the head and down along the back of your back. This gives the experience a more circular feeling and may be easier for some people.

These variations are not extremely different in their practical function which is to draw awareness away from the physical senses and inward to the spinal flow, but one of the four small variations may be easiest for you to work with at your present level.

Whole Body Up

In this variation you draw the energy widely up through the whole body rather than focusing on the spine at all. You exhale down in the same manner. You may still use the mulabandha and others as necessary. While this lacks the precision of the other variations it can be very effective in awakening movement and easier to visualize.

Whole Body Down

This is simply the opposite of the previous.

All of these visualizations and gentle physical movements can have a very positive effect on your energy body. With each of them conduct the kumbhaka segment exactly as in the beginning of this section. You will notice the difference.

Conclusion

We have explored a lot of territory in this small book, and you may want to read it over a few times. However, the whole essence of the thing can be summed up in a few more words.

Seek to experience your meditation object with every part of awareness leaving aside every part of your personal self.

Enlightenment is seeing reality without the filters of ego. Meditation is focusing the mind in such a way that this seeing is possible.

Imagine being totally okay, not wishing anything was any better than it is right now. You are in tune with the whole universe and there are no problems even conceivable.

Imagine not craving for anything, no addiction, no obsession, no desire. Instead you just feel absolutely happy with just how things are.

Imagine not disliking anything or anyone. Imagine not being worried about the future. Imagine not being sad about the past. You are just totally and genuinely joyous.

Imagine not believing a bunch of pointless things about yourself or others. Imagine just experiencing what is without any value judgement or labels, and just being ecstatically happy.

Imagine having unshakable calmness, equanimity, tranquility and focus.

True awareness is the direct experience of what we already know to be true. The universe is just a bunch of subatomic particles bouncing off of each other with no single one of them any more important than any other.

And remember that I have created a series of audio recordings based upon the instructions in this book so if you want to make the process incredibly easy you can just go grab one of those recordings and get started right now.

www.ingramcontent.com/pod-product-compliance
Lightning Source LLC
Chambersburg PA
CBHW021015090426
42738CB00007B/797